NEUROSCIENCES:
The Basics

Contributors

Dade T. Curtis, M.A., M.S.

Stanley Jacobson, Ph.D.
Tufts University
College of Medicine
Boston, Massachusetts

Elliott Marcus, M.D.
Saint Vincent Hospital
Worcester, Massachusetts

Gerald Palagallo, M.D.
Methodist Medical Center
Peoria, Illinois

NEUROSCIENCES:
The Basics

Brian A. Curtis, Ph.D.
University of Illinois
College of Medicine
at Peoria
Peoria, Illinois

Lea & Febiger
Philadelphia   London   1990

Lea & Febiger
200 Chester Field Parkway
Malvern, Pennsylvania 19355-9725
U.S.A.
1-800-444-1785

Lea & Febiger (UK) Ltd.
145a Croydon Road
Beckenham, Kent BR3 3RB
U.K.

Library of Congress Cataloging-in-Publication Data

Curtis, Brian A.
    Neurosciences : the basics / Brian A. Curtis ; contributors, Dade
  T. Curtis . . . [et al.].
        p.   cm.
    Includes bibliographical references.
    ISBN 0-8121-1309-8
    1. Neurology.   2. Neurophysiology.   I. Curtis, Dade T.
  II. Title.
    [DNLM: 1. Nervous System—anatomy & histology.   2. Nervous System—
  physiology.   3. Nervous System Diseases.   WL 100 C9775n]
  RC346.C874   1990
  616.8—dc20

PRINTED IN THE UNITED STATES OF AMERICA

Print No.   4   3   2   1

P R E F A C E

From an integrated neurosciences course at Tufts Medical School taught by Elliott Marcus, M.D., Stanley Jacobson, Ph.D., and myself, two books have evolved, both using the problem solving approach. An *Introduction to the Neurosciences* (originally published by W.B. Saunders in 1972; the second edition will be published by Lea & Febiger) is a text suitable for medical students, with the three of us as coauthors. References in this book to *An Introduction to the Neurosciences* may be to either edition.

This book—a text suitable for graduate nursing, occupational and physical therapy students, and other allied health students and workers—developed more slowly; however, it owes a substantial debt to *An Introduction to the Neurosciences*. It began as a workbook for physician assistant students at Northeastern University, was expanded for occupational therapy students at the University of Illinois at Urbana, and was perfected over the last few years for graduate nursing students of the University of Illinois College of Nursing here in Peoria. To all of the students who have used the earlier versions of the book and contributed to its development, thank you!

The problem-solving approach is used extensively in both the text, in a section at the end of each chapter, and in Chapter 10. The use of case histories for problem solving owes much to the example set by my colleague, Elliott Marcus. Instructors may obtain answers either from Lea & Febiger or from me. I would like to hear from you.

I am grateful to my clinical colleagues for encouraging my interest in clinical neuroscience and making patient contact possible; I have talked with each of the persons whose case I describe. I am particularly grateful to three clinical chiefs, the late John Sullivan, M.D., of New England Medical Center Hospitals; Frank Iber, M.D., now at Loyola Medical Center; and Pat Elwood, M.D., here in Peoria, for their help and encouragement. It is a pleasure to acknowledge the help of Evelyn Hodgkins here in Peoria, Ken Bussy and Tom Colaiezzi of Lea & Febiger, and Lilliane Chouinard of Editing, Design & Production with the multitude of steps between my ideas and this finished book.

Brian A. Curtis
UICOMP
Box 1649
Peoria, IL 61656

CONTENTS

1

Introduction to the Nervous System

How the brain functions has baffled and intrigued observers for centuries. It was clear to the ancients that the brain was the seat of thought and behavior. To satisfy their curiosity, they began dissecting the brain and speculating on the activities of its various parts. Scientific inquiry over the last 300 years has revealed a great deal about the human nervous system and the localization of functions within the various structures of the nervous system. Recent developments such as computed tomography (CT), magnetic resonance imaging (MRI), and positron emission tomography (PET) allow detailed study of the living brain and contribute to a greater understanding of the brain's functions and more precise localization of disease processes.

The nervous system can be considered at several levels of anatomic and functional complexity. We should never forget that the different anatomic parts work together to integrate the purposeful actions of the complete nervous system. The two basic anatomic divisions of the nervous system are the *peripheral nervous system* (PNS) and the *central nervous system* (CNS). The CNS consists of the brain and spinal cord. The PNS consists of nerves leading to and from the CNS and connects the central nervous system to the rest of the body. Lying primarily outside the bony structures of the skull and vertebral column, the peripheral nervous system will be discussed in Chapter 2.

Completely encased in the skull and vertebral column (Fig. 1-1), the CNS forms the integrative and thinking portions of the nervous system. Because human actions and dreams originate in the CNS, we will begin our discussion in this area.

CENTRAL NERVOUS SYSTEM

The central nervous system consists of the spinal cord, which lies within the vertebral column, and the brain, which lies within the skull (Fig. 1-1).

Spinal Cord

The spinal cord serves the body below the shoulders by providing sensory

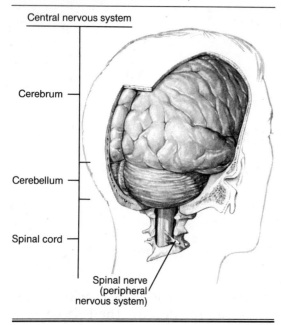

Central nervous system

Cerebrum

Cerebellum

Spinal cord

Spinal nerve
(peripheral
nervous system)

The brain stem is a direct continuation of the spinal cord and shares many of the spinal cord's functions. Size and functions of the brain stem have changed very little with the evolution of vertebrates. The brain stem serves three major functions: (1) it is a connecting link between the cerebrum, the spinal cord, and the cerebellum; (2) it provides the face and neck with sensory and motor functions via the cranial nerves; and (3) it is a center of integration both for the cranial nerves (e.g., the eye blink reflex and for several visceral functions, such as control of heart and respiratory rates. The cerebellum is a coordinator of the voluntary muscle system. It acts together with the brain stem and cerebrum to maintain balance and to provide harmonious muscle movements. The staggering gait that results from excessive alcohol intake is due primarily to the selective depression of cerebellar function.

and motor function via the peripheral nerves. Sensory function is achieved by the carrying of nerve impulses from receptors to the spinal cord; motor function is achieved by the carrying of nerve impulses from the spinal cord to muscles and glands. The spinal cord is the connecting link between the brain and the body and is a lower level center for the integration of sensory and motor activity. For example, the classic knee-jerk reflex is completed within the spinal cord.

LOCALIZATION OF CEREBRAL FUNCTION

The cerebrum occupies a special, dominant position in the human CNS. Most of the functions of the nervous system with which you are familiar are conscious ones located in the cerebrum, where the final integrative or "conscious" actions occur. We will, therefore, concentrate first on the cerebrum, for in man the cerebrum dominates all other parts of the nervous system; it is impossible to discuss the functions of these parts without referring to the cerebrum. Once we understand something about cerebral structure and function, we can discuss the spinal cord and other parts of the brain in more detail.

Brain

The brain consists of three major parts: the *brain stem*, the *cerebellum*, and the *cerebrum*. The cerebrum is by far the largest part of the human brain. It occupies the upper portion of the cranium and consists of separate right and left hemispheres. Inferior to (beneath) the cerebrum lie the brain stem (hidden in Fig. 1-1) and the cerebellum.

The cerebrum is a paired structure, with right and left *cerebral hemispheres.* Each hemisphere governs actions in the opposite side of the body. For example, voluntary movements of the right hand are "willed" in the left cerebral hemisphere.

Each hemisphere consists of several layers. The outer layer is composed of a dense collection of nerve cells called *gray matter*. This outer layer, about 1 cm thick, is called the *cerebral cortex* and is molded into *gyri* (ridges) and *sulci* (valleys). The deepest sulci are termed *fissures*. The deeper layers of the hemisphere consist primarily of axons and are called *white matter* because of the glistening white myelin around the axons.

Lateral Surface

The cerebrum is divided by the lateral fissure (Fig. 1-2), which runs on the lateral surface of the cerebrum from the open end in front, posteriorly, and dorsally (backwards and up). The lateral fissure defines a tongue of cerebrum ventral to it, the *temporal lobe* (Fig. 1-2).

Temporal Lobe. The primary auditory cortex is a major area in the temporal lobe. It receives auditory impulses from the auditory receptors in the inner ear. The *primary auditory cortex* is localized on the *transverse temporal gyrus*, which is located at the posterior and dorsal margin of the temporal lobe buried on the inner slope of the lateral fissure. To see the transverse temporal gyrus, we must reflect (pull) the temporal lobe out and down. When a recording electrode is placed on this gyrus during neurosurgery, a large and characteristic electrical response follows when noise is played into a patient's ear (Fig. 1-3). If a weak current is passed into a stimulating electrode placed in this same location, conscious patients report "hearing" tones or noise. The primary auditory cortex, then, is an excellent example of a region of cortex that has a well-defined function.

In right-handed individuals, the left temporal lobe surrounding the trans-

F I G U R E 1-2
The left cerebrum showing the lateral fissure, the superior boundary of the temporal lobe. (From *An Introduction to the Neurosciences.*)

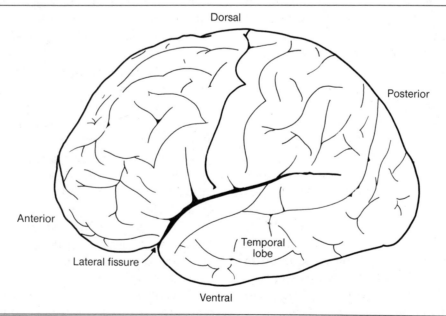

F I G U R E 1-3
An evoked cortical potential from the transverse temporal gyrus in response to a sound in the ears. (From *An Introduction to the Neurosciences*.)

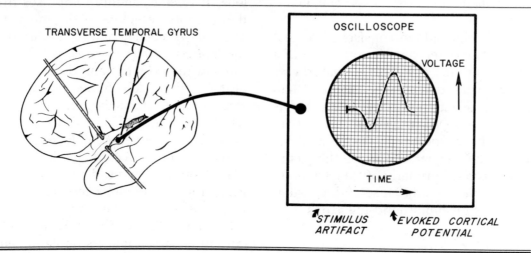

verse temporal gyrus is involved in more complex interpretation of auditory signals. If the cells of this area die, patients are not able to interpret sounds as words. The cells on the homologous surface of the right hemisphere may be involved in musical discrimination. A person who cannot understand spoken language may still join you in singing "Happy Birthday." The functions of the rest of the temporal lobe, particularly the anterior tip, are more difficult to specify, but storage of long-term memory is one of them.

Frontal Lobe. The frontal lobe is defined by the lateral fissure inferiorly and the *central sulcus* posteriorly. The central sulcus is a major landmark of the cerebral cortex (Fig. 1-4) but is not as prominent and unvarying a landmark as is the lateral fissure. The central sulcus runs over the convexity of the hemisphere to the lateral fissure. There are usually two well-formed and continuous gyri on either side of this sulcus; it takes some experience to be able to pick out the central sulcus.

The gyrus immediately anterior to the central sulcus is the *precentral gyrus* (Fig. 1-5), which functions as the *primary motor cortex*. From this gyrus, signals descend through the brain stem to the spinal cord in the *corticospinal* tract and, after one or more synapses, travel out through the peripheral nervous system to control muscles. Destruction (a lesion) of part of the precentral gyrus causes paralysis on the opposite side of the body.

Further anterior in the frontal lobe is an area called the *premotor cortex* (Fig. 1-5). Here more complex motor movements such as speaking and throwing a ball are organized. The premotor cortex is a larger area and is not readily definable in terms of gyri. Its anterior border is vague. The anterior and the inferior portions of the frontal lobe are involved in control of emotional behavior. These areas, referred to as the *prefrontal cortex* (Fig. 1-5), appear to have an inhibitory function predicated on the future consequences of present actions. Patients who have disease in the prefrontal cortex or who have undergone prefrontal lobectomies (removal of the lobes) often have

F I G U R E 1-4
A photograph of the left brain showing the boundaries of the frontal lobe. (Courtesy of
S. Jacobson, Ph.D.; from *An Introduction to the Neurosciences.*)

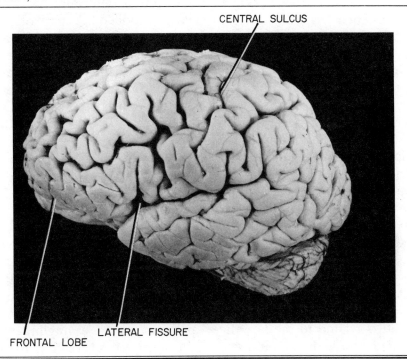

F I G U R E 1-5
The right brain. The precentral gyrus is the origin of commands for voluntary strength
and motion of specific muscles on the opposite side of the body.

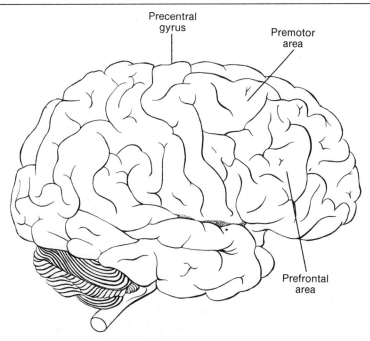

little awareness of the social consequences of their actions. For example, such patients may not realize others would object to their urinating on the floor in a crowded bus station.

Parietal Lobe. Immediately behind the central sulcus lies the parietal lobe (Fig. 1-6). Its anterior boundary is the central sulcus. The ventral boundary is the lateral fissure or a line continuing in the same direction. Its posterior boundary is poorly defined on the lateral surface. Several component areas of the parietal lobe may be distinguished. Immediately posterior to the central sulcus is the *postcenteral gyrus* (Fig. 1-6), the *primary sensory cortex* that receives impulses from the sensory receptors in the skin. Each small area along the postcentral gyrus is related to a particular part of the body: the medial end is related to the leg, the center is related to the hand, and the end next to the lateral fissure is related to the face. We can "feel" pain, touch, and

pressure at lower levels of the nervous system, especially in the brain stem, but we cannot determine where the stimulus is applied. A patient who loses a small portion of the hand area of the left postcentral gyrus can perceive when a pin is stuck into his right hand but cannot tell or show the examiner where the pin was placed.

Perception of a cotton strand drawn over the hairs on the back of the hand is an example of a sensory modality subserved exclusively by the postcentral gyrus. If a recording electrode is appropriately placed on this gyrus during a neurosurgical procedure, cortical responses can be elicited by stroking the hairs of the back of the contralateral hand, that is, the hand on the opposite side of the body. If a stimulus is applied through the same electrode, conscious patients report a tingling sensation in the contralateral hand. If the postcentral gyrus is destroyed by a pathologic process, patients cannot feel the cotton

F I G U R E 1-6
The left cerebrum showing the major boundaries of the parietal lobe. The postcentral gyrus receives primary sensation from the opposite side of the body.

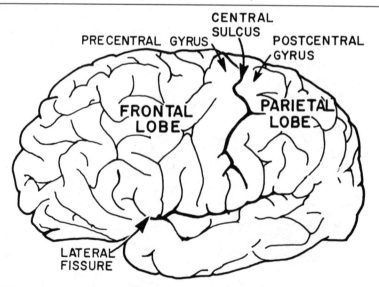

wisp. Functions of the remaining portion of the parietal lobe include sensory discrimination of a higher order, such as recognizing a number drawn on the palm of the hand or being aware of the opposite side of the body. A patient with a lesion in the posterior parietal lobe will often forget to button the contralateral cuff of his shirt.

Stroke

Loss of blood supply to all or part of the brain is the most common cause of the sudden loss of neural functions and is a leading cause of disability and death.

CASE HISTORY
Ischemic Stroke

N. L. is a 58-year-old, right-handed white carpenter. While watching the fights on TV with several of his friends, he suddenly slipped, unconscious, out of his chair to the floor. He regained consciousness a few minutes later but was unable to move his left side. When examined in the emergency room he had a left hemiparesis (paralysis of the left face, arm, and leg) and a total left sensory loss; he could not feel even deep pain on the left side.

He was admitted for observation. He quickly regained the ability to tell if he was stuck with a pin but was unable to localize the place where the pin touched the skin. He received daily physical therapy and had a strong will to regain mobility. During the next 4 weeks voluntary control returned to the face, shoulder, and leg as did all sensation to these areas. Three months after the "shock" he was able to walk slowly. His left arm was held in a flexed position across his chest. Six months after the shock he could get around well but still could not use his left hand. In this case a large area of cortex was deprived of blood and did not function; however, only a small area was totally destroyed. The portion of the precentral

gyrus controlling hand movement and the portion of the postcentral gyrus perceiving fine sensory function never recovered.

Medial Surface

When the cerebral hemispheres are cut apart at the midline and the hemispheres separated, all four lobes are seen extending onto the medial surface (Fig. 1-7).

Occipital Lobe. The occipital lobe is most easily seen on the medial surface. The tissue on either side of the *calcarine fissure* in the occipital lobe is the *primary visual cortex*. Light flashed into the eye evokes electrical signals from electrodes placed over this area of the cortex or on the scalp above it. The remainder of the occipital lobe lies on the lateral surface of the cerebrum and is involved in interpreting and categorizing visual sensations. The interpreting and cataloging functions of the occipital lobe that relate to language take place only in the *dominant hemisphere*. The dominant hemisphere is on the left for 97% of the population, for all right-handed individuals and for half of those who are the left-handed.

A prominent structure on the medial surface of the cerebrum is the *corpus callosum* (Fig. 1-7). This wide band of nerve fibers interconnects the two cerebral hemispheres and transfers information between them. Immediately above the corpus callosum is the *cingulate gyrus*. This area is involved in emotional reponses. It functions in conjunction with other regions of the brain such as the frontal lobe and areas of the brain stem.

The cingulate gyrus illustrates one of the difficulties in studying the nervous system, which evolved slowly with phylogenetically newer structures dominating the functions of older structures. In

F I G U R E 1-7
A sagittal section that separates the two cerebral hemispheres and bisects the brain stem and cerebellum. The corpus callosum interconnects the two cerebral hemispheres. (Courtesy of S. Jacobson, Ph.D.; from *An Introduction to the Neurosciences*.)

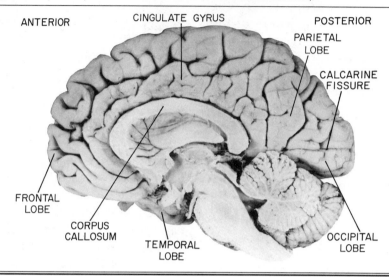

other words, the cingulate gyrus is dominated by the newer frontal lobe and in turn it dominates the even older brain stem structures. The older structures did not, however, disappear as evolution proceeded, and their presence complicates the study of the nervous system. This layering of increasingly complex functions affords enormous opportunity for rehabilitation after damage. It challenges us to find ways for voluntary commands to reach these lower structures through alterntive pathways.

CELLS OF THE CENTRAL NERVOUS SYSTEM

Neurons

Neurons are the active cells of the entire nervous system, for they carry its signals and transact its business. Each neuron has a central *cell body* from which radiate many threadlike processes. Numerous receiving processes, called *dendrites*, carry nerve signals to the cell body. A single process, the *axon*, carries nerve signals away from the cell body.

At its termination the axon branches extensively to form *synapses* with other neurons. The minute space across which a nerve impulse passes from an axon of one neuron to stimulate the dendrites of other neurons is called a *synaptic junction*. At the synapse, packets of a chemical *neurotransmitter* are released from the axon in response to a nerve impulse traveling down from the cell body. The neurotransmitter diffuses across the narrow gap to the dendrite of the adjoining neuron. There the neurotransmitter combines with a specific region of the dendrite's membrane and passes on the information contained in the nerve impulse.

In the simplest synapses, only one neurotransmitter is released by an axon and is then quickly destroyed. The junction between the axon of a motor neuron and skeletal muscle is an example. The neuron signals "jump," and the muscle contracts once. In the brain, most axons release several neurotransmitters. Some are not destroyed immediately and influence neuronal behavior for hours, maybe days, and are called *neuromodulators*. Neurons are usually influenced by several neurotransmitters and neuromodulators. Many drugs interact with neurotransmission and neuromodulation.

Dendrites. The dendrites of a neuron in the precentral gyrus (Fig. 1-8A) fan out over the ⅜-inch thickness of the white matter of the cerebral cortex and make perhaps 10,000 synaptic contacts with axonal processes. At these synapses, every conceivable type of information (sight, smell, and sense of position to name a few) are conveyed. The synapses are characterized by vesicles of a chemical neurotransmitter in the presynaptic terminal of the axon and a thickening of the postsynaptic (dendritic) membrane. Dendrites transfer information from the synapse to the cell body by a passive electrical process, which, like light from a light bulb, weakens the further it travels. Hence synapses close to (or on) the cell body exert greater influence over the cell body than do those at the far end of the dendrite.

Cell Body. The cell body of every neuron includes a DNA-containing *nucleus* and a dense collection of organelles (Fig. 1-8B). Rod-shaped *mitochondria* contain the enzymes that generate energy for the cell by oxidative degradation of glucose. Nerve cells have a much lower capacity for anaerobic metabolism than do most cells of the body. They are very dependent on a constant supply of glucose and oxygen from arterial blood. Most of the cytoplasm of the neuron cell body is

occupied by tubular membraneous canals called the *endoplasmic reticulim*. *Ribosomes* attach to these canals to form the rough endoplasmic reticulum or Nissl substance. Ribosomes are full of messenger RNA and produce proteins. The *Golgi apparatus* manufactures secretory vesicles that participate in cell membrane formation and in repair throughout the neuron. *Lysosomes* engulf worn out cell components, break them down, and eject the debris from the cell.

Axon. One axon arises from each cell body. Each axon contains a rich collection of neurotubules and neurofilaments (Fig. 1-8C). These tubules and filaments transport enzymes produced by the rough endoplasmic reticulum down to the synaptic regions where they produce the neurotransmitters.

Where the axon leaves the cell body it forms a specialized integrating region, the axon hillock. Here, all signals pouring into the nerve cell body through its many dendritic connections are summed and the decision is made whether to transmit one or more action potentials. If the answer is yes, a signal is sent from the brain down the 2 or 3 feet of axon to the spinal cord and signals, for example, "dorsiflex the great toe." Just beyond the axon hillock the *myelin sheath* (Fig. 1-8D), characteristic of all large (5 to 15 μm) axons, begins. This sheath forces the action potential to jump from one *node of Ranvier* to the next, thereby increasing the conduction velocity.

The extensive branching of the axon when it emerges from the descending corticospinal tract occurs in about ¼ inch of spinal cord and may influence 2,000 to 3,000 neurons in the spinal cord.

After neuronal death, microglia engulf and digest (phagocytize) the dead cells, which leaves a space that slowly fills with fibrous tissue. The central ner-

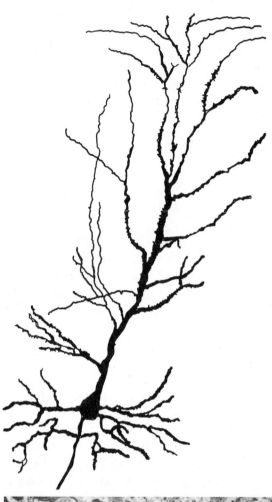

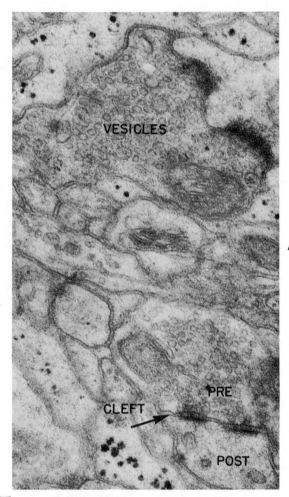

VESICLES

PRE

CLEFT

POST

A

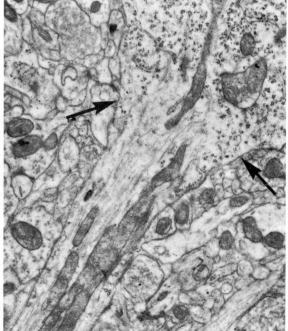

C

F I G U R E 1-8
A pyramidal cell *(upper left)* with electron
micrographs of the dendritic tree **(A)**, cell
body **(B)**, and axon hillock **(C)** in the
precentral gyrus. The axon joins the
corticospinal tract and crosses the neuroaxis
at the brain stem-spinal junction. The
myelinated axon **(D)** emerges from the
descending corticospinal tract *(opposite page,
lower right)* to influence the neurons which
run into the peripheral nervous system to
stimulate skeletal muscles to contract.
(Electron micrographs in **A, B,** and **C** courtesy
of S. Jacobson, Ph.D., from *An Introduction
to the Neurosciences.* Electron micrograph in
D courtesy of R. Caughey, M.S., University
of Illinois College of Medicine at Peoria.)

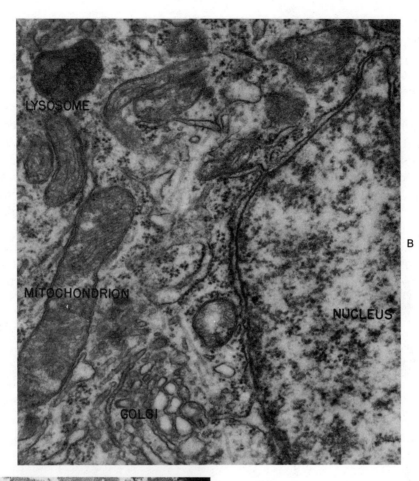

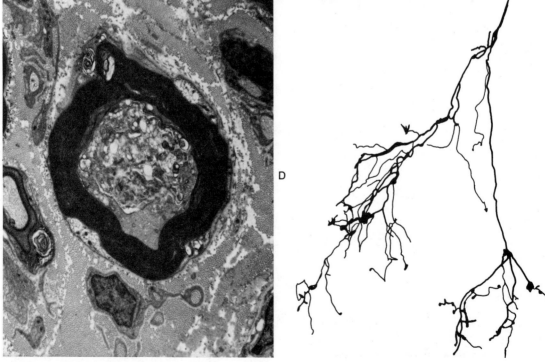

vous system has, unfortunately, very little or no power of regeneration, largely because neurons have lost the ability to divide. Consequently neoplasms (cancer) of central nervous tissue are uncommon.

Even the ability of CNS axons and dendrites to regrow is limited. Axons or dendrites cut off from the cell body degenerate. Research is progressing slowly on the uses of embryonic nerve growth factors to promote axonal and dendritic regrowth in adults. Patients can often regain functions destroyed in a cerebral cortical stroke, always by using surviving structures lower in the nervous system such as the brain stem or spinal cord.

Glial Cells

Glial cells are specialized connective tissue cells that support neurons both structurally and functionally. *Oligodendrocytes* produce the myelin sheaths of axons and form other close connections with neurons. If the oligodendrocyte dies, so does the axon. *Astrocytes* form a barrier between the neurons and blood vessels (Fig. 1-9). Many chemicals that easily enter the extracellular spaces around the other cells of the body cannot enter the extracellular spaces around neurons or influence their behavior. This concept of a restricted space is called the *blood-brain barrier*, and astro-

F I G U R E 1-9
The principal glial cells of the CNS surrounding a pyramidal cell (*P*) of the precentral gyrus. The astrocytes (*A*) wrap around blood capillaries (*C*), nerve cells (*P*), and synaptic junctions (*S*). Oligodendrocytes (*O*) form the myelin sheaths of axons.

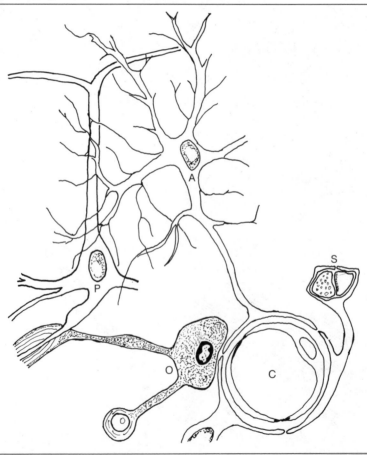

cytes play a major role in its formation. Astrocytes send out long processes that wrap around synapses and presumably regulate the composition of the synaptic gap. Astrocytes surround neurons and support them both anatomically and metabolically.

Unlike neurons, glial cells can divide during adult life because they are connective tissue, not nervous tissue. This ability to divide makes them susceptible to uncontrolled cell division termed *neoplasia* or cancer. Most tumors of the CNS are glial in origin. Astrocytomas, oligodendromas, and glioblastomas, (tumors of a common stem cell) are examples of CNS glial tumors. Meningiomas (tumors of the coverings of the brain) are also common. Tumors usually cause a loss of function that is minor at first but which gets progressively and steadily worse. The rate of loss is variable; glioblastomas grow quickly and function is lost in a matter of weeks, while meningiomas grow slowly, often for years.

POST-TEST

Locate and label the following structures on Figures 1-10 and 1-11 (see p. 14):

Lateral fissure
Precentral gyrus
Central sulcus
Postcentral gyrus
Frontal lobe
Parietal lobe
Temporal lobe
Occipital lobe
Primary auditory cortex
Primary visual cortex
Primary motor cortex
Corpus callosum
Area destroyed in Norman L.'s stroke
Area initially nonfunctional in Norman L.'s stroke

CASE HISTORIES

A case history contains many clues both to the location and to the type of disease causing that individual's disabilities. In the following case histories you should identify the disability and link that disability to a structure within the nervous system. Try to find a single location within the nervous system where the structures you have identified come in close approximation. Once you have identified the location of the disease process, use the clues to speculate about the disease type.

1. Your classmate has gradually had more difficulty understanding both the teacher and her classmates. She can hear sounds and indeed continues to play the piano by ear, but she makes frequent mistakes when reading written poetry aloud. She has no difficulty in responding when writing the answer to a written question but often makes mistakes when writing answers to spoken questions. Which portion of her nervous system is not functioning properly?

2. Some years ago a medical student who had been wounded in the head during the Vietnam War challenged me to find his neurologic deficit. Muscle strength was fine, as was coordination. Sensory discrimination was intact except for diminished ability, compared to the right side, to tell me which way his left toes were moving. Sensory discrimination on the right side appeared intact, however. Numbers drawn on the sole of the student's right foot were easily recognized, but when numbers were drawn on the sole of his left foot, he could only guess. What region of this student's central nervous system was destroyed?

F I G U R E 1-10
The lateral surface of the cerebrum.

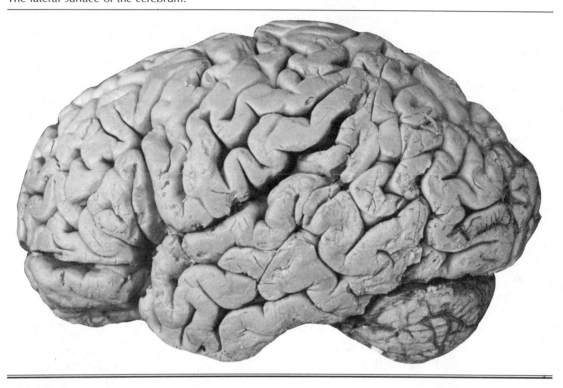

F I G U R E 1-11
The medial surface of the brain.

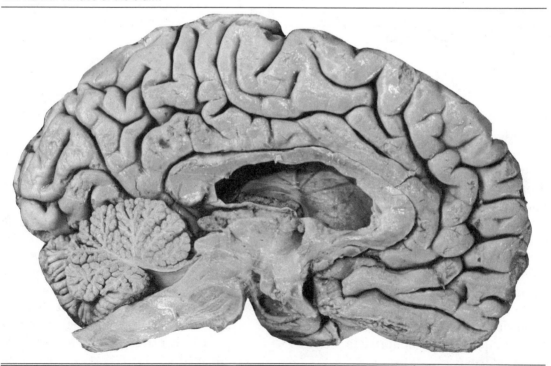

2

Nerve and Muscle

NEURON PHYSIOLOGY

Neurons (See Fig. 1-8) are the active cellular units of the nervous system. Neuronal membranes have some very intriguing properties, and mastering these properties is basic to an understanding of the integrative action of the nervous system. This section concentrates on membrane properties common to all parts of the neuron as well as on those special membrane properties that enable the axon to conduct action potentials.

Cell Membrane

The cell membrane delimits all cells. It is the boundary separating the sodium- and chloride-rich extracellular fluid from the potassium- and protein-containing intracellular fluid. The cell membrane is composed of lipids arranged as a bimolecular leaflet (Fig. 2-1). The lipids are arranged so that the nonpolar, water-insoluble portion of the molecule faces the center of the membrane while the polar, water-soluble parts face the inner and outer edges of the membrane. The membrane edges are in contact with the aqueous solutions of the extracellular and intracellular fluid compartments. The outside of the membrane is covered by a thin layer of protein. The total cell membrane is about 4 to 5 nm thick. The cell membrane also contains a fascinating array of membrane-spanning proteins. It is these membrane-spanning proteins that confer special properties to different cells.

MEMBRANE VOLTAGE

All neurons and most other cells maintain a negative intracellular voltage. It is as if a cell had a little battery across its cell membrane. This "battery" maintains the negative voltage between the interior and exterior of the cell and derives its energy from the potassium gradient across the cell membrane. Cells contain a high concentration of potassium ($K_i = 140$ mM), while the extracellular fluid contains a low concentration ($K_o = 3$ mM). The cell membrane can transform energy in the form of a chemical gradient of an ion into energy in the form of an electric voltage difference by mechanisms we will discuss presently.

F I G U R E 2-1
A drawing of the phospholipid bilayer that comprises the bulk of the cell membrane.
The lipid-soluble tails face each other while the more water-soluble heads face the
extracellular fluid and the cytoplasm. Most membranes are covered with a thin protein
skin.

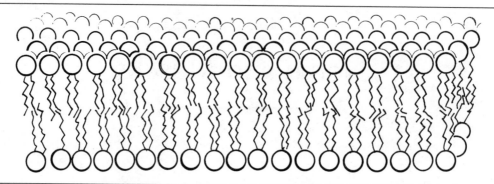

A pure-lipid bilayer membrane would not allow potassium to move across the membrane because potassium ions are insoluble in lipid. Yet soon after radioactive potassium is added to the extracellular solution, neurons are found to contain radioactive potassium. When these neurons are returned to a nonradioactive solution, the radioactivity leaves the neurons. The cell membrane is clearly permeable to potassium ions (K^+), which move through the cell membrane.

Potassium Channels

Potassium ions move through specialized protein channels in the membrane (Fig. 2-2). These channels can be isolated, indentified, and incorporated into

F I G U R E 2-2
A drawing of a potassium channel inserted in a lipid bilayer. *S* represents the selectivity
filter that discriminates between potassium and other ions. *G* represents a gate that
opens and closes the channel. The dotted sphere represents the control function of the
gate. Many different types of control have been described including transmembrane
voltage, intracellular Ca^{2+}, and extracellular neurotransmitters.

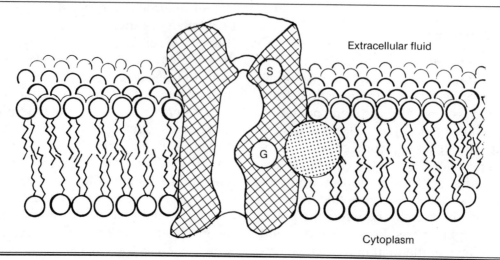

artificial membranes to recreate the properties of the living cell membrane. A recording from such a channel (Fig. 2-3A) shows that the channel opens and closes rapidly and frequently. This particular channel was open about 25% of the time.

These channels are selective for potassium. In Figure 2-3B, the solution inside the membrane was changed from a K^+-rich solution to one containing rubidium (Rb^+). Even though K^+ and Rb^+ are very similar, the number of ions flowing through the channel dropped dramatically. Most transmembrane channels are specific for the ion that they allow to pass when they are open.

Most cells contain several thousand potassium channels on their surface. It is very difficult with a 0.1 μm pipette to find a place on the membrane with only one channel. On the statistical basis, then, a large number of these channels are open at any one time and provide a sizable pathway for potassium ions to move down their concentration gradient. Yet the potassium ion concentration of cells remains constant and the potassium flux leaving the cells is small. Why, with a sizable pathway and an equally sizable *concentration force* (from the 140 mM/3 mM potassium gradient), doesn't potassium rush out of the cell?

This question is answered once you realize that potassium ions are positively charged. Negative charges exist predominantly on the intracellular proteins, which do not move around and certainly cannot leave the cell. Hypothetically, before any potassium channels open, you would find an equal number of positive and negative charges inside the neuron and consequently no voltage difference across the cell membrane. When a potassium channel opens, a K^+ from inside the neuron moves into the open potassium channel, down its concentration gradient. The K^+ leaves behind a negative charge on the protein fixed inside the cell; there is a net surplus of one negative charge inside the cell, and the inside of the cell becomes ever-so-slightly negative. As more and more positively charged potassium ions start down the potassium concentration gradient through open potassium channels in the membrane, the interior of the cell becomes increasingly more negative.

As the inside of the cell becomes slightly negative, a second force, *electro-*

F I G U R E 2-3
A recording of ions passing through a single potassium channel. **(A)** The fluid facing the cytoplasm surface contained K^+, and many ions traversed the channel each time it opened. **(B)** When Rb^+ was substituted for K^+, the number of ions crossing through the channel was reduced even though the channel opened as often as before. (Patch-clamp method; data adapted from Findley, I. *J. Physiol.* 350:179–195, 1984.

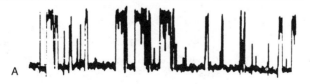

static attraction, begins to work between the positive charge on the potassium ion and the negatively charged interior of the neuron. This attraction acts to hold potassium ions within the cell. In less than a second an equilibrium is established between the *concentration force*, which tends to move potassium down its concentration gradient out of the cell and the *electrostatic force*, which attracts the positively charged potassium ions back into the negatively charged cell. This equilibrium results in a stable voltage of about 0.1 volt (100 mV), inside negative, across the resting cell membrane of all nerve and muscle cells. Only about 0.005% of the intracellular potassium moves into the membrane channels—and stays there—to establish this equilibrium voltage. Because this is an equilibrium, once the potassium-protein complex is generated within the cell, the voltage is maintained without the further expenditure of energy.

This equilibrium between an electrostatic (voltage) force and a chemical concentration force is described quantitatively by the *Nernst equation*. Now wait! Before you panic, I am just saying in symbols what we agreed was happening:

$$\frac{\text{Electrostatic}}{\text{force}} = \frac{\text{Concentration}}{\text{force}}$$

$$zFV_K = -RT \log K^+{}_i/K^+{}_o$$

or, rearranging

$$V_K = -RT/zF \log K^+{}_i/K^+{}_o$$

where V_K is the voltage across the membrane, R and F are constants, and z is the valence of the potassium ion ($+1$), while T is the temperature and $K^+{}_i$ and $K^+{}_o$ are the potassium concentrations inside and outside the cell. For potassium ions at 20°C (68°F), this equation becomes

$$V_K = -58 \log 140 \text{ mM}/3 \text{ mM}$$
$$= -97 \text{ mV}$$

Translating back into English, this equation says that the voltage we can expect from a potassium concentration gradient is proportional to the ratio of ionic concentration. If $K_o{}^+$ increases and $K_i{}^+$ remains constant, then the concentration ratio decreases and the expected equilibrium voltage is less negative. Often, V_K is termed the *potassium equilibrium voltage*. At this voltage and concentration ratio, K^+ is an equilibrium across the cell membrane.

Resting Membrane Voltage

The actual negative voltage measured in resting cells is called the resting membrane voltage. Experimental values of a single muscle cell are shown in Figure 2-4. I choose a muscle cell to show that many types of cells have the same basic properties. These experimental values are well described by the Nernst equation, which assumes that potassium is the only permeant ion. Because the resting membrane voltage closely approximates the potassium equilibrium voltage, the potassium ion is an equilibrium across the resting membrane.

We find voltages across the membranes of most types of cells. Most of these voltages can be described to a first approximation by the Nernst equation for potassium. These voltages range from -65 mV to -90 mV; the membrane is said to be polarized. When discussing changes in the actual membrane voltage of a cell, the term *depolarize* denotes a movement to more positive voltages (i.e., -90 to -60 mV) and *hyperpolarize* denotes movement to more negative voltages (i.e., -90 to -110 mV). We use the convention that the extracellular solution is 0 millivolts.

F I G U R E 2-4
The relation between the external potassium
concentration and the resting membrane voltage.
As the external potassium increased, the voltage
across the membrane decreased. (From Hodgkin,
A.L., and Horowicz, P.: *J. Physiol.* 148:127–160,
1959.

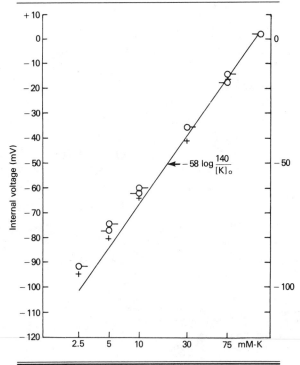

charged ion. Indeed, the *sodium equilibrium potential* calculated from the Nernst
equation is

$$V_{Na} = +58 \log 120 \text{ mM}/20 \text{ mM}$$
$$= +45 \text{ mV}$$

Only a voltage of +45 mV inside the cell
would bring Na^+ into electrochemical
equilibrium across the membrane if Na^+
were the only permeant ion. In a cell
with a resting membrane voltage of −90
mV, sodium ions, if permeable to the
membrane, are 135 mV away from equilibrium; this 135 mV difference is a significant force drawing Na^+ into the cell.
Because there are both electrical and
concentration forces acting on Na^+, we
call this 135 mV difference an *electrochemical gradient*.

Actual neuronal membranes are
about 100 times more permeable to potassium ions than to sodium ions. Each
time a positive sodium ion manages to
sneak into the cell, the cell becomes a little less negative. A potassium ion is now
liberated from the constraints of electrostatic attraction and escapes from the
cell. Remember, the only force holding
K^+ inside the cell was the negative internal voltage. If the voltage is less negative, some K^+ can leave. Because of this
continual small Na^+ leak into the cell,
the membrane voltage is a little less negative than that predicted by the potassium equilibrium voltage. Figure 2-4
shows that at K_o of 2.5 and 5 the experimental voltage points are less negative
than predicted by the Nernst equation.
This is true of most cells because most
cells leak a little sodium.

Thus we have the idealized situation
described by the Nernst equation in
which K^+ is the only permeable ion. Potassium ions enter the membrane channels and stay there, held in an equilibrium between electric and chemical
forces. This is an equilibrium that re-

Sodium Leakage

The preceding discussion assumed that
the membrane was permeable only to
potassium ions because it contained
only potassium-selective channels. Real
cell membranes do not reach that degree
of perfection. Neuronal membranes are
also permeable to sodium ions (Na^+).
Radioactive sodium ions enter and leave
cells slowly. A little Na^+ enters through
K channels. The rest of the Na^+ enters
through the Na channels we will consider a little later.

That sodium ions enter cells from the
extracellular fluid should be no surprise,
for the Na concentration gradient (Na_i =
120 mM and Na_o = 20 mM) is into the
cell and the negative interior voltage of
the cell is very inviting to a positively

quires no further expenditure of energy. Contrast this equilibrium with the real-life situation for most cells, which have a Na$^+$ leakage into the cell. This Na$^+$ leakage allows K$^+$ to escape from the constraints of the equilibrium, to exit the channel, and to leave the cell. To maintain a constant intracellular environment, Na$^+$ must be transported out and K$^+$ transported into the cell; this requires the expenditure of energy.

Active Transport

Just as it is clear that sodium ions move down an electrochemical gradient into the cell, any sodium ion movement out of the cell must be up an electrochemical gradient. This movement requires energy, an active transport with ATP as the energy source. The active transport of sodium out of cells has been studied extensively, and the membrane-spanning protein responsible has been isolated. In all cells, a little sodium leaks in and a little potassium leaks out; active transport keeps the internal levels of potassium high and sodium low. About 10% of our resting metabolic rate is consumed with Na$^+$/K$^+$ active transport.

ACTION POTENTIALS

Each axon is a long cylinder that, when activated, can carry a stereotyped electrical message from cell body to synaptic region. This electrical message is called an action potential. Like most cells, the axon maintains a negative resting membrane voltage derived from the potassium ion gradient (-70 mV in Fig. 2-5).

F I G U R E 2-5
Voltage traces from a cat spinal cord neuron showing the response to two stimuli, one at subthreshold **(A)**, and the other at threshold **(B)**. Stimulus *B* induced an action potential, a transient reversal of membrane polarity, from the threshold voltage (-53 mV) to $+20$ mV. (From Schwindt, P., and Crill, W.: *J. Neurophysiol.* 43:1296 –1318, 1980.)

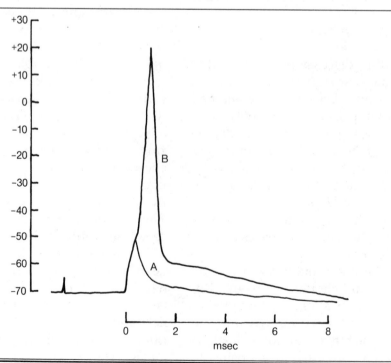

Whenever the axon is stimulated, the voltage across the membrane becomes positive and within 1 msec returns to the resting membrane voltage (Fig. 2-5A). This sudden reversal of polarity (electric sign) from -70 to $+20$ mV is called an action potential. No matter where on the axon it is measured, the duration and amplitude are the same.

Sodium Channels

The peak positive voltage of the action potential decreases as external Na^+ decreases (Fig. 2-6). As the sodium equilibrium voltage decreases, so does the peak voltage. The positive voltage of the ac-

tion potential is derived from the sodium equilibrium potential, which is normally $+45$mV. Sodium ions are suddenly and briefly able to move down their electrochemical gradient through open Na channels in the membrane. The sodium ions carry excess positive charge into the axon, and the voltage across the membrane becomes positive: -70 to $+20$ mV. Sodium channels open rapidly in response to a stimulus, allow Na^+ to move into the cell, and then close quickly.

While many different types of stimuli generate action potentials, all depolarize the axon membrane to a critical voltage, *threshold*, that opens sodium channels and generates an action potential. The stimulus that produced Figure 2-5A is subthreshold. A stimulus just 0.1 mV more positive initiated an action potential (Fig. 2-5B). Some force, external to this patch of axon membrane, does work on this patch of axon membrane to depolarize the axon from the resting membrane voltage (-70 mV in this case) to the threshold voltage of -53mV. At threshold, sodium channels open transiently, and the sodium equilibrium voltage briefly dominates the membrane.

In Figure 2-7A, individual records of a single sodium channel show that the channel usually opens in response to a depolarizing stimulus. Only rarely does the channel remain open for 10 to 15 msec. Most often the channel opens for 5 mesc, and sometimes the channel does not open. Sodium channels occupy about 1% of the axon surface area. It is the average response of many hundreds of open sodium channels that is responsible for the action potential we record. The average response can be obtained by summing either many sodium channels reacting to a single stimulus or by recording one sodium channel reacting to many stimuli.

F I G U R E 2-6

The effect of low-sodium solutions on the action potential. Records *1* and *3* were taken with the squid axon in normal sea water. Record *2A* was taken with the axon in ⅓ seawater and ⅔ dextrose; *2B* was taken in ½ seawater and ½ dextrose. Note that the peak voltage of the action potential was reduced in 2.

V_{Na} for 1 and 3 $= 58 \log 460/50 = +56$ mV
V_{Na} for 2A $\quad = 58 \log 153/50 = +28$ mV
V_{Na} for 2B $\quad = 58 \log 230/50 = +38$ mV

(From Hodgkin, A.L., and Katz, B.: *J. Physiol.* 108:37–77, 1949.

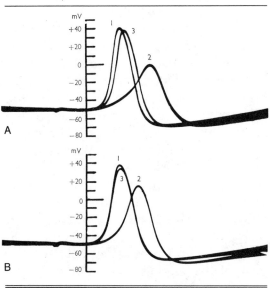

F I G U R E 2-7
(A) Opening of a Na channel in response to a depolarization from −100 mV to −25 mV for 30 msec. Notice the variability in response. If the channel opens, it usually does so soon after the depolarization. **(B)** The summed response (on a different time scale) of 144 consecutive depolarizations like the ones in **A**. The average response is a rapid opening followed by closing; half the time, the channel closes within 5 msec. (From Patluka, J., and Horn, R.: J. Gen. Physiol. 79:333−351, 1982, by copyright permission of the Rockefeller University Press.)

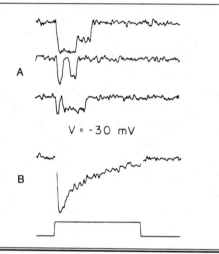

Figure 2-7B is the average of 144 responses to the same depolarizing stimulus and shows a sudden increase in the probability that sodium channels will be open immediately after depolarization to or below threshold. Indeed most of the sodium channels open after a threshold stimulus. The probability of being open falls rapidly and then remains low, but not zero, as long as the depolarization continues. The same pattern pertains to the hundreds of sodium channels present in any patch of axon membrane.

Open sodium channels permit sodium ions to move down their electrochemical gradient into the cell and to carry excess positive charges into the cell. The peak rate of influx can be calculated as 150 Na$^+$ per millisecond per channel. The first few sodium ions entering Na channels displace potassium ions from K channels and allow K$^+$ ions to move down their concentration gra-

dient, out of the cell. The rest of the sodium ions bring excess positive charges into the membrane and cause the voltage across the cell membrane to become positive. Because the sodium channels do not remain open for very long, as we saw in Figure 2-7B, the membrane voltage returns to its resting (−70 mV) level quickly. The closing of the sodium channels is called *inactivation*.

The Na$^+$ selectivity filter is on the outside of the channel and is the site of attachment of a number of naturally occurring paralyzing toxins, including tetrodotoxin (TTX). These toxins prevent Na$^+$ ions from entering the channel and altering the voltage across the membrane. Local anesthetics enter the channel, bind, and place the channel in a long-lasting refractory state.

Action Potential Propagation

The preceding discussion was concerned with the properties of a single patch of membrane near the tip of the recording electrode. The mechanism by which the action potential spreads down the axon is simply current spread from the active to the inactive regions (Fig. 2-8). The voltage of the active region is very close to the sodium equilibrium voltage, whereas the voltage of the resting region, a little further down the axon, is close to the potassium equilibrium voltage. Ions will flow between these two regions of unequal voltage. When the ionic flow crosses the membrane of the resting region, it depolarizes the membrane to threshold and increases sodium permeability. This results in further depolarization and in the generation of an action potential in this previously resting region. This process continues down the axon. As can be seen in Figure 2-8, there is a short time delay between the peak of the action potential at A and B. The conduction velocity of *nonmyelinated* axons varies from 0.3 meters per second

F I G U R E 2-8
The spread of activity by local current flow from an active region to a resting region.
The conduction velocity is Δx/Δt.

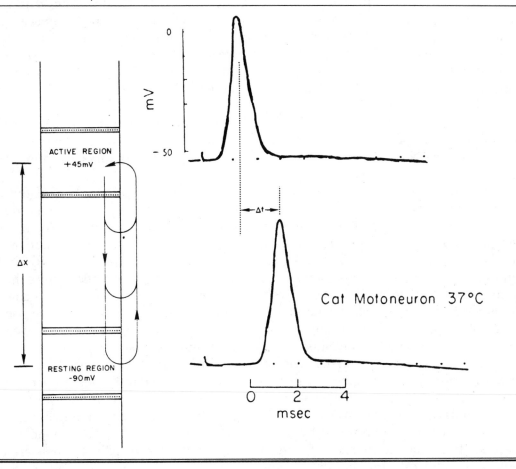

for a 0.7 μm axon to 25 meters per second for a 500 μm giant axon.

Conduction in Myelinated Axons

In unmyelinated axons, increased conduction velocity is achieved by increasing the diameter of the axon. Nature has found another way to achieve increased conduction velocity: by increasing the distance between active regions along the axon. The time between successive peaks of the action potential is little affected by the distance between the active regions. Consequently, conduction velocity increases as the distance between active regions increases. The myelin sheath around many axons prevents ions from moving across the membrane, and therefore only the spaces between successive myelin sheaths, the nodes of Ranvier, are available for ionic movement. As a result, the action potential jumps from node to node, about 1 mm at a jump. Conduction velocities in myelinated axons run from 10 meters per second for a 2 μm axon to 100 meters per second for a 20 μm axon.

Refractory Period

Immediately after an action potential, axons are incapable of carrying a second action potential because the Na channel is inactivated. This period lasts for about the duration of the action potential, 1 to

2 msec. This absolute refractory period is followed by a relative refractory period during which a supranormal stimulus is necessary to evoke an action potential. This period lasts for another 2 to 3 msec. These two refractory periods put an upper limit of the neurons's frequency response at about 200 per second.

CALCIUM CHANNELS

Calcium channels are another major component of the membrane of excitable and contractile cells. Most cells maintain very low Ca_i^{2+}. The calcium equilibrium voltage, V_{Ca}, is ~ + 100 mV. Unlike sodium, which carries charge across the membrane and then needs to be actively transported out of the cell, calcium has a dual role, both as a depolarizing charge carrier and also as an intracellular messenger. Ca^{2+} entry depolarizes cells on the way through the membrane, just as Na^+ does, and then activates a vast array of intracellular processes. Contraction, for example, is controlled by intracellular free calcium, some of which enters through calcium channels in the membrane. Calcium channels are intriguing because there are many types and because many clinically useful blockers have been discovered.

NEUROMUSCULAR JUNCTION

As motor axons of peripheral nerves enter skeletal muscle, each axon branches upwards of 200 times; each branch innervates a single muscle cell, also called a muscle fiber. All muscle fibers innervated by a single motor axon are called a *motor unit* and contract together. The degree of branching and the number of muscle fibers innervated by a single motor axon determine the sensitivity of the

motor unit. An extraocular unit of six muscle fibers has much finer control of movement than does an antigravity muscle of the leg with 200 muscle fibers.

The junctional region between an axon and a skeletal muscle consists of the presynaptic axon terminal, and synaptic cleft, and the postsynaptic membrane of the muscle fiber (Fig. 2-9). This area is often called the end-plate region. It has the same components as does a synapse between an axon and a dendrite.

The presynaptic ending of the axon is filled with vesicles containing the transmitter acetylcholine (ACh), mitochodria to supply energy, and an enzyme system to make the acetylcholine. When an action potential enters the presynaptic region of the axon, Ca channels open. Then Ca^{2+} enters the region and accelerates the release of acetylcholine from the presynaptic terminal.

The released acetylcholine diffuses across the synaptic cleft to activate the muscle membrane. The postsynaptic membrane is rich in channels that open when exposed to acetylcholine (Fig. 2-10). When these ACh channels are open they allow the passage of all small ions, particularly Na^+ and K^+, which depolarize the membrane and set up an action potential on the muscle surface, which induces contraction.

The postsynaptic membrane contains the enzyme acetylcholinesterase, which cleaves acetylcholine and renders it inactive. Consequently, the acetylcholine released by the presynaptic terminals enters a competitive arena. Will it bind to a receptor before it is rendered inactive? The esterase also pulls ACh off the receptor and as a result, the end plate is briefly depolarized.

The entire process is very rapid. An end plate is depolarized for a very short time. The end result is that one action potential from an axon induces one ac-

F I G U R E 2-9
An electron micrograph of a human neuromuscular junction (end plate). Structures
include the nerve terminal *(Ne)* and components of a skeletal muscle fiber: a nucleus
(Nu), the receptor containing membrane *(Re)*, and the sarcomeres of contractile protein
(Sa). (Courtesy of U. Kalyan-Raman, M.D., and R. Caughey, M.S., University of Illinois
College of Medicine at Peoria.)

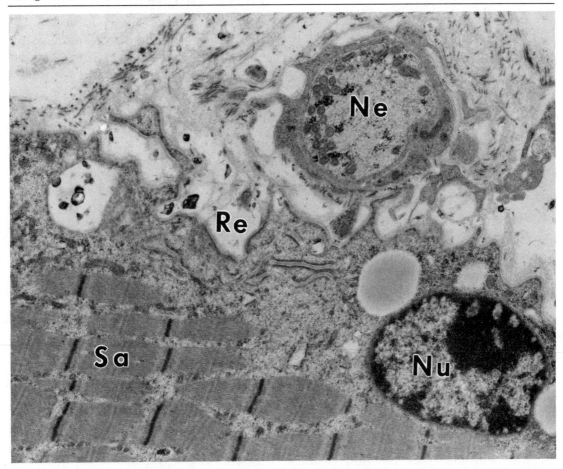

tion potential in a muscle fiber, and the
muscle fiber contracts.

Myasthenia gravis is a disease of the
neuromuscular junction characterized by
progressive muscular weakness during
activity. If the affected muscle is a flexor
of the hand, the first squeeze of a ball is
forceful, but the next few rapidly decrease in power; after a dozen squeezes,
hardly any power is left. Strength returns after the patient rests. The condition is diagnosed by a characteristic
history and by improvement with anticholinesterase therapy. Edrophonium
(Tensilon), a short-acting drug that
must be injected, is used for diagnostic
purposes. Neostigmine, pyridostigmine
(Mestinon), and ambenonium (Myte-
lase) can be given orally and have obvious advantages for long-term therapy.
The dosage and schedule must be
worked out for each patient and will
change from time to time.

Myasthenia gravis is an autoimmune
disease; antibodies are produced by the
body against the acetylcholine receptors
of the muscle end plate. The antibodies
cover a fair fraction of the available re-

F I G U R E 2-10

Recordings of a single acetylcholine (ACH) receptor channel. Acetylcholine channel complimentary DNAs were introduced into a mouse fibroblast; ACH channels were synthesized by the fibroblast and inserted into the cell membrane, which previously had no ACH channels. 2μM ACH was added to the bath 5 sec before the second trace. Acetylcholine induced the channel to open more often and for longer periods of time. (From Claudio, T., et al.; *Science* 238:1688–1693, 1987. Copyright 1986 by the AAAS.)

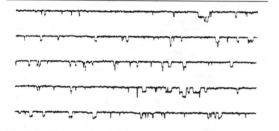

ceptors of the neuromuscular junction and make ACh-receptor interaction, hence muscle contraction, less likely. Anticholinesterase therapy allows released ACh to remain in the synaptic cleft longer and increases the probability of released ACh reacting with an ACh receptor. Longer-term therapy to ameliorate the autoimmune process includes thymectomy, prednisone, and plasmapheresis.

The neuromuscular junction is the site of action of many naturally occurring substances. *Botulin toxin* prevents relase of acetylcholine from the axon terminal. By attaching to the ACh receptor on the muscle membrane many snake and spider venoms prevent attachment of acetylcholine and hence block nerve-muscle junction transmission. Curare, discovered by the South American Indians, acts in the same way.

Other drugs such as succinylcholine are used during surgery to produce paralysis by inactivating the action potential on the muscle membrane. Many insecticides cause paralysis and death by blocking nerve-muscle junction trans-

mission by the inactivating acetylcholinesterase.

SKELETAL MUSCLE

Our bodies contain many anatomically separate skeletal muscles, which are connected to bones and other structures by tendons. Each is made up of muscle fibers that run from one tendon to the other. The entire length of the muscle is often 1 or 2 feet. Since muscles can only contract, an intricate system of opposing lever systems allows each joint to both flex and extend.

Muscle Structure

The striated structure of skeletal muscle has been very thoroughly studied and is summarized in Figure 2-11. The individual muscle fibers are 100 to 150 μm in diameter and up to one-half meter long, among the largest cells of the body. Muscle fibers are made up in turn of cylindrical *myofibrils,* about 1 μm in diameter. The characteristic banded pattern of skeletal muscle, alternating dark *A bands* and light *I bands,* can also be seen in myofibrils. The I bands are made up of thin filaments of *actin,* which meet in a centrally located *Z line.* The distance between Z lines is a *sarcomere.* The A band is composed of thicker filaments of the enzyme *myosin.*

Myosin converts the chemical energy of ATP into mechanical energy when it interacts with actin. During contraction, this energy is used to slide the actin filaments past the myosin filaments. This shortens the sarcomere length and hence the length of the muscle fiber. Both thick and thin filaments are arranged in hexagonal arrays with the thin filaments slipping through the spaces between the thick filaments.

F I G U R E 2-11
Each skeletal muscle fiber is made up of long, cylindrical myofibrils **(D)** showing a
repeating pattern of dark A bands and lighter I bands. The I bands are bisected by a
darker Z line. At higher magnification **(E),** the thin actin filaments of the I band and the
thick myosin rods are clearly seen. Bridges project from the myosin rods to make
tension generating connections with actin filaments. In cross section (**F** through **I**), each
set of filaments is in a complementary hexagonal array. (Drawing by Sylvia Colard
Keene from Bloom and Fawcett: *A Textbook of Histology.* Philadelphia. W.B. Saunders,
1968.)

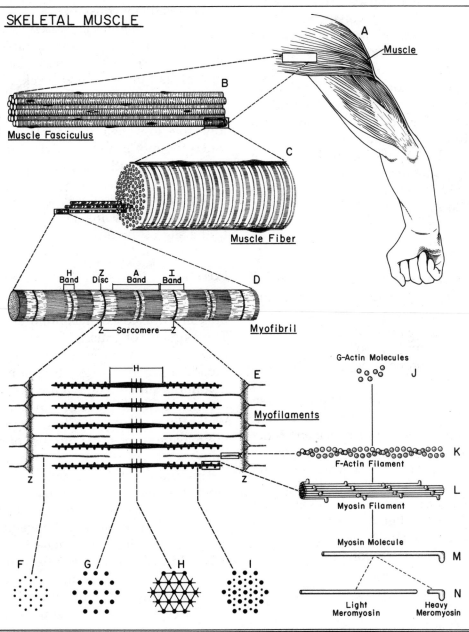

Tension

Tension is generated when thin and thick filaments overlap, and *actomyosin bridges* are formed. Figure 2-12, shows three major phases of the *length-tension relationship* of skeletal muscle. In very highly stretched muscle (Fig. 2-12B), the filaments barely overlap; very little tension is produced because very few bridges can be formed. As the muscle is allowed to shorten, more actomyosin bridges are formed and tension increases. When all of the possible bridges are formed (Fig. 2-12C), tension is at a maximum. As the muscle shortens further (Fig. 2-12D), the opposing ends of the actin filaments begin to overlap, interfere with bridge formation, and cause tension to decline.

Excitation-Contraction Coupling

The events between the action potential of the surface membrane and the chemical interaction of the actomyosin bridges are described as excitation-contraction coupling. Inpocketings of the surface membrane brings the electric activity of the surface into the depths of the fiber along each Z line. These inpocketings make contact with Ca-containing sacks, the sarcoplasmic reticulum. Activation at the surface membrane results in Ca^{2+} release into the filament lattice. Actomyosin bridge formation, hence contraction, is catalyzed by Ca^{2+}. Soon after its release, Ca^{2+} is transported back into the sarcoplasmic reticulum and contraction ceases.

Atrophy

The size and strength of each muscle group are dependent on two factors: (1) the amount of exercise the muscle receives regularly and (2) the existence of an intact motor nerve. Atrophy describes a decrease in the bulk of a muscle accompanied by a loss of strength. *Disuse atrophy* occurs when a limb is immobilized in a cast or paralyzed by a cerebral stroke. Disuse atrophy may reduce the muscle bulk by 10% to 30% in 2 or 3 months time. The bulk then remains relatively constant.

Denervation atrophy, caused by loss of the motor nerve, is a very rapid and striking process. The muscle may lose 50% of its bulk in a few weeks. Hence when assessing muscle strength and bulk, it is important to decide how rapidly the loss has taken place. Often when the motor nerve is dying, it sends out action potentials that cause a couple of hundred muscle fibers to twitch. This twitching or *fasciculation*, can often be seen and gives valuable information as to the site of the disease process.

Exercise

Weight lifting results in greater muscle bulk and increased maximum strength. The number of muscle fibers does not increase, but their volume does. Each muscle fiber has a greater number of myofibrils and greater amounts of the contractile proteins actin and myosin. Weightlifters also learn how to activate the maximum possible number of motor units.

Endurance athletes, such as long-distance runners and swimmers, increase their maximum rate of oxidative metabolism without significant change in muscle bulk. This increase occurs in several ways. Individual muscle fibers increase their capacity for oxidative metabolism by generating additional enzymes, usually 2 to 4 weeks after beginning endurance exercise. The O_2 delivery system is enhanced with an increased number of blood capillaries, increased strength of the heart, and augmented capacity of the lung. Improved neuromuscular co-

F I G U R E 2-12
The length tension curve **(A)** and electron micrographs **(B, C,** and **D)** of skeletal muscle showing the overlap of the sliding filaments. When the filaments barely overlap **(B),** tension is low. When all bridges are attached **(C),** tension is maximum. When the thin filaments overlap **(D),** tension declines. (Data from Gordon, A. F., Huxley and Julian, F. J.: *J. Physiol.* 184:170–192, 1966. Electron micrographs courtesy of Brenda Eisenberg, Ph.D., University of Illinois College of Medicine, Chicago, IL.)

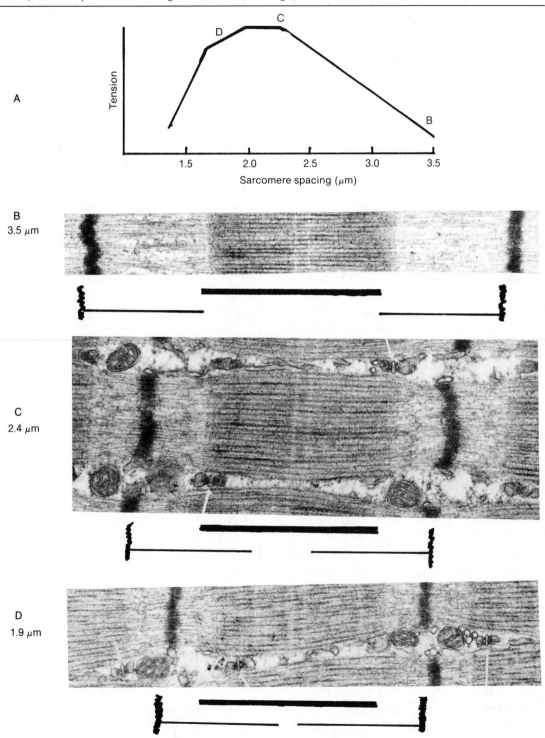

ordination is an important part of their training.

Duchenne type muscular dystrophy occurs almost exclusively in males and is inherited as a sex-linked, recessive trait. More than half the cases begin before the boy is 3 years old, and nearly all occur by age 10. The muscles of the pelvic girdle are affected first. Their weakness leads to clumsiness in walking, frequent falling, and difficulty in climbing stairs and in getting up from the floor. The disease progresses rapidly so that 5 years after its onset the child is confined to a wheelchair. The disease usually spreads to the shoulder girdle as well. The prognosis for the patient is poor, and death by heart or respiratory failure usually occurs 15 to 20 years after the onset. The heart is often involved in the pathologic process. The muscles of affected individuals lack the membrane assembly protein dystrophin, presumably because of a defect or absence in the gene that codes for it. The general location of the gene has been found. A newly developed model of the disease in mice will help us immensely in finding suitable therapy.

PERIPHERAL NERVOUS SYSTEM

The peripheral nervous system (PNS) consists of all nervous tissue outside the bony structures of the vertebral column and skull. There are two major divisions—the voluntary and the autonomic nervous system. The autonomic nervous system is involved in activities such as blood pressure regulation and gastrointestinal motility.

The voluntary portion of the PNS has the major functions of carrying sensory information into the central nervous system (CNS) by sensory nerves and carrying motor commands out to the muscles by motor nerves. In general,

motor and sensory nerves run together in nerve trunks. Since the spinal cord is the most common destination or origin of these nerve signals, this chapter includes some information about spinal cord function; more will be presented in the next chapter.

Primary Sensory Modalities

The English language contains a rich collection of words for describing the interplay of the world on our skin. Several hundred words exist that describe pain alone. For clinical and physiologic purposes, however, we try to define and divide these sensory stimuli more carefully. They are commonly divided into five categories: (1) nociceptive (damaging), (2) pain and temperature, (3) vibration and conscious position sense, (4) unconscious position sense, and (5) light touch. Each of these modalities has a specific sensory receptor that responds to it exclusively.

Nociceptive stimuli are those capable of causing tissue damage and usually are not tested. Crushing and burning are among the nociceptive stimuli.

Pain and temperature share the same receptors, which are easily and harmlessly stimulated by the light touch of a pin. Be sure to test several places on each limb so you adequately test these receptors and their pathways through the spinal cord to the upper brain stem, where we "feel" these stimuli. The pathway to the contralateral postcentral gyrus must be intact for us to localize the stimulus (to tell where it occurred), such as the dorsal side of the left thumb. *Numbness* is a sensation generated high in the CNS when the pain and temperature receptors of an area of the body "have not been heard from" for a time. The "pins-and-needles" sensation resulting from a crossed leg is an example.

Vibration receptors and pathways are tested by placing the base of a heavy, vibrating tuning fork on the bony prominences of the ankles, knees, fingers, and elbows. *Conscious position sense* is tested by an examiner moving a joint and asking the patient which way it was moved.

Unconscious position sense relates to the cerebellum; touching a finger to the nose tests both this pathway and the cerebellum.

Light touch is tested by drawing a wisp of cotton or an artist's paint brush lightly over the skin.

Pathway to the Spinal Cord

The axons that leave the sensory receptors come together to form the *peripheral nerves.* Peripheral nerves also contain motor axons to the muscles of each region. There are three major peripheral nerves of the arm. The *radial nerve* generally supplies the muscles and skin of the upper arm and the medial forearm. The *median nerve* generally supplies the muscles of the forearm as well as the thumb and first two fingers. The *ulnar nerve* supplies the intrinsic (situated within) hand muscles and the last two fingers. Ulnar nerve sensory distribution is often unintentionally tested when the "funny bone" on the back of the elbow is struck. The specific areas of the skin supplying receptor nerve fibers to each of these peripheral nerves are shown in Figures 2-13 and 2-14.

The *femoral* and *obturator* nerves supply the muscles and skin of the upper thigh. The *sciatic nerve* supplies the rest of the leg.

Sensory information is carried in the nerves by the action potentials we have discussed. The intensity of the stimulus is signaled by how many action potentials pass along the nerve each second.

As these great nerve trunks approach the spinal cord, they come together to form great tangles of nerves or *nerve plexi.* Each plexus is turn sends *spinal nerves* into the *spinal canal.* The sensory and motor fibers of each peripheral nerve enter and leave the spinal cord by several spinal nerves. The specific entry of axons of the median nerve through the spinal nerves C6, C7, C8, and T1 is shown in Fig. 2-15A. Conversely, the C7 spinal nerve supplies or receives axons from several peripheral nerves, including the radial and the median (Fig. 2-15B).

Once inside the spinal canal, the spinal nerves divide and enter the spinal cord (See Fig. 3-1). All the sensory axons enter through the *posterior root,* while all of the motor axons leave the spinal cord by way of the *anterior root.* Once inside the spinal cord itself, the nerve fibers carrying the separate sensory modalities form bundles or tracts and take varying and devious pathways to the contralateral postcentral gyrus, which will be discussed in Chapter 3.

Sensory Distributions

The only spinal cord lesion that destroys all the sensory modalities from a region of the body is a complete transaction of the spinal cord, usually obvious on other grounds. The absence, then, of *all* sensory modalities from a limited region of skin is ample cause to consider a lesion of a peripheral pathway. This is especially true when loss of muscular control (paralysis) is also present in the same area. There are two different locations for a lesion in a peripheral pathway, a peripheral nerve or a spinal nerve/root. Each interrupts different groups of sensory and motor axons.

F I G U R E 2-13
Comparison of dermatome and peripheral nerve innervation of the skin: an anterior
view. (Courtesy of Marc Bord, M.D., from *An Introduction to the Neurosciences.*)

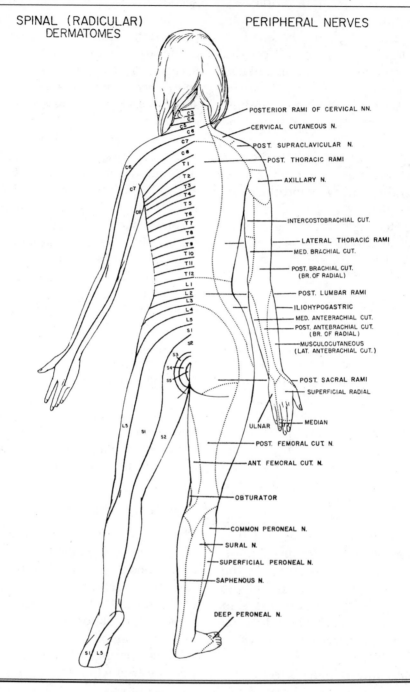

SPINAL (RADICULAR)
DERMATOMES

PERIPHERAL NERVES

POSTERIOR RAMI OF CERVICAL NN.

CERVICAL CUTANEOUS N.

POST. SUPRACLAVICULAR N.

POST. THORACIC RAMI

AXILLARY N.

INTERCOSTOBRACHIAL CUT.

LATERAL THORACIC RAMI

MED. BRACHIAL CUT.

POST. BRACHIAL CUT.
(BR. OF RADIAL)

POST. LUMBAR RAMI

ILIOHYPOGASTRIC

MED. ANTEBRACHIAL CUT.

POST. ANTEBRACHIAL CUT.
(BR. OF RADIAL)

MUSCULOCUTANEOUS
(LAT. ANTEBRACHIAL CUT.)

POST. SACRAL RAMI

SUPERFICIAL RADIAL

ULNAR

MEDIAN

POST. FEMORAL CUT. N.

ANT. FEMORAL CUT. N.

OBTURATOR

COMMON PERONEAL N.

SURAL N.

SUPERFICIAL PERONEAL N.

SAPHENOUS N.

DEEP PERONEAL N.

F I G U R E 2-14
Comparison of dermatome and peripheral nerve innervation of the skin: a posterior
view. (Courtesy of Marc Bord, M.D., from *An Introduction to the Neurosciences*.)

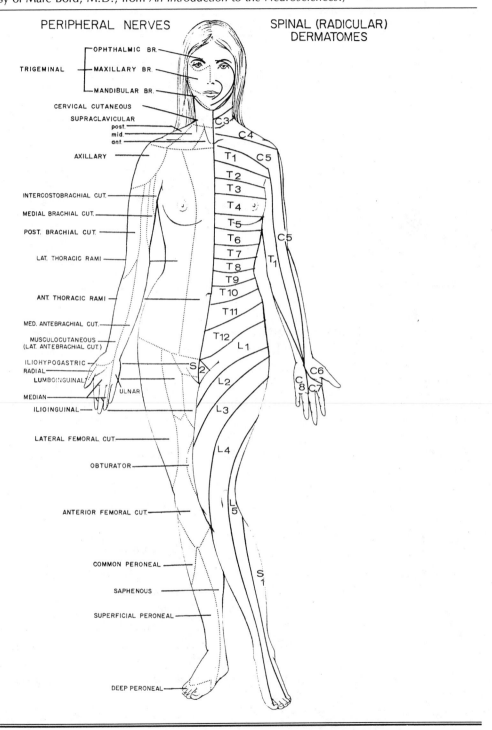

F I G U R E 2-15
The brachial plexus is a tangle of axons connecting peripheral nerves of the arm with spinal nerves. **(A)** Axons to and from the median nerve enter the spinal cord by spinal roots C6, C7, C8, and T1. **(B)** Axons using the C7 spinal nerve to enter or leave the spinal cord distribute to the radial, musculocutaneous, and median nerve.

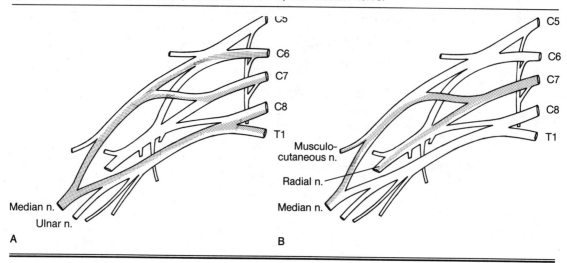

Peripheral nerve loss gives characteristic sensory loss patterns as shown on the left sides of Figures 2-13 and 2-14. A complete sensory loss of the first two fingers is most likely the result of median nerve injury.

Many types of pathology can compress nerves and cause loss of function. Nerves are very sensitive to pressure and lack of oxygen. Frequently peripheral nerves are pinched as they go through tunnels (e.g., the carpal tunnel of the wrist) or grooves in bones (e.g., the radial groove of the humerus). Loss of or damage to blood supply is a common cause of nerve function loss. Most of us are familiar with the numbness associated with crossing our legs; the femoral artery is compressed, little blood flows, nerve conduction stops, and higher centers warn us of danger by referring the sensation of numbness to the ischemic limb.

Spinal nerve / posterior root damage results in the second sensory map shown on the right sides of Figures 2-13 and 2-14. That region of skin, all of whose sensory receptor axons enter the spinal cord by a single spinal nerve or posterior root, is known as a *dermatome*. Important dermatomal boundaries are C5, shoulders; C8–T1, hand, back of arm; T10, umbilicus; and L5 and S1, ankle, back of leg. Dermatome and peripheral nerve boundaries are sometimes very similar and difficult to distinguish. Nevertheless it is important to do so since the site and types of pathology differ.

Motor Innervation

Skeletal muscles also have two innervation patterns, spinal nerve and peripheral nerve. Segmental motor innervation, tabulated in Tables 2-1 and 2-2, follows much the same distribution as the sensory nerves, although most muscles are innervated by more than one anterior root or spinal nerve.

Peripheral Neuropathy

This is a fairly common symptom of an underlying disease process. There is a

T A B L E 2-1
Segmental motor innervation: upper extremity.

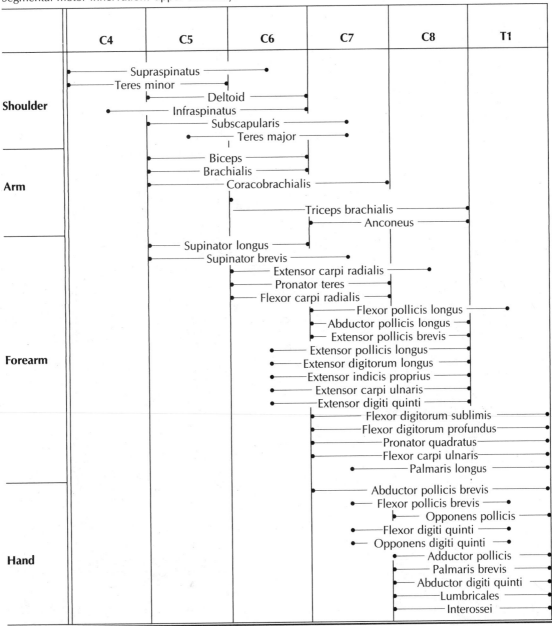

characteristic slow loss of sensation over the hands and feet, called a stocking-and-glove distribution. The patient is frequently not aware of the loss. All sensory modalities are usually involved, but not equally, and there is often loss of the motor pathways to the muscles, hence voluntary weakness.

C A S E   H I S T O R Y
Peripheral Neuropathy

E.S. is a thin, alert 79-year-old white male. His ability to perceive the vibration of a tuning fork is absent at both ankles and markedly diminished at the knees and hands. The fork had to be struck very hard for him to feel it, and he

T A B L E 2-2
Segmental motor innervation: lower extremity.

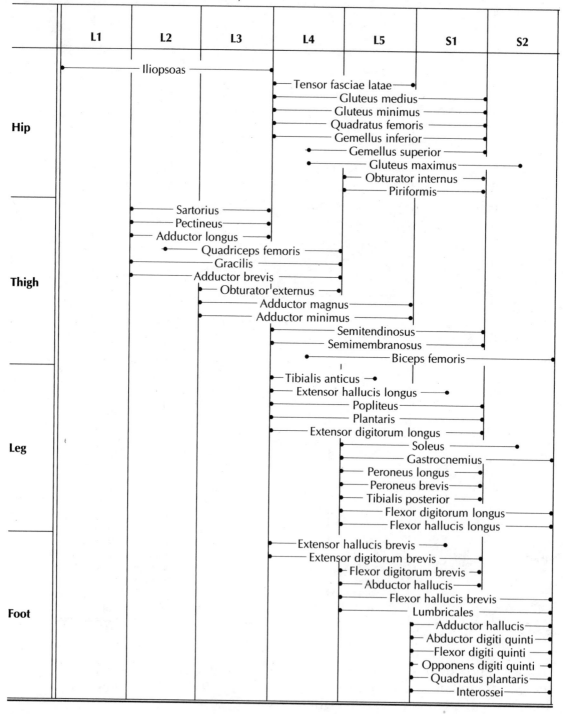

could no longer feel it at vibrations at which the examiner could. His ability to tell which way his fingers and toes were moved (position sense) was also diminished; on large amplitude movements, changes were perceived but errors in direction were made. The ability to "feel" a pinprick was absent in the feet and diminished in the hands. Perception of light touch (stroking the skin with a wisp of cotton) was diminished in his right hand and arm and over the entire left leg. Muscle strength was diminished in his hands. He was very unsteady in walking.

Peripheral neuropathy is a sign of many diseases. It is important to find the disease and treat it so that the progression of nerve death may be stopped. Uremia, (E.S.'s problem), untreated diabetes, alcoholic vitamin deficiency, and heavy metal poisoning are common causes.

A peripheral neuropathy of rapid onset is the Guillain-Barre syndrome with motor nerves ususally more affected than sensory nerves. The muscle weakness begins in the feet and rises so that ultimately respiration is difficult. If patients are suspected of having this disorder, they should be closely followed and a respirator should be immediately accessible to them. Most patients achieve complete recovery.

POST-TEST

1. Define potassium equilibrium voltage and resting membrane voltage.

2. If the Na^+ leak into cells could be plugged, how would you expect the resting membrane voltage to change?

3. If serum (extracellular) potassium increases from 3 mM (normal) to 8 mM (hyperkalemia), how will the resting membrane voltage change (hyperpolarize, depolarize)?

4. (The following data are from Creutzfeld, D. D., et. al.: Electroencephalogs Clin Neurophysiol 15:508–519, 1963.)

   a. A group of normal persons have a K_i of 150 mM and K_o of 3 mM. What is the potassium equilibrium voltage? (Because body temperature is 37°C, use $V_K = -61 \log K_i/K_o$.) The resting membrane voltage is -81 mV. Why are they different?

   b. A rare disease, familial periodic paralysis, causes occasional muscle paralysis. Muscle fiber K_i is 150 mM and does not vary during attacks. When these patients are strong, their $K_o = 4$ mM. What is the expected V_K? The measured value is -68 mV. Why might it be different from V_K?

   c. When these patients are paralyzed, $K_o = 7$ mM. What is V_K? The resting membrane voltage is -46 mV. Why is it so low?

   d. Why do these patients become paralyzed?

5. During acidosis, hydrogen ions (H^+) move into muscle cells in exchange for K^+. If K_i becomes 120 mM and K_o becomes 10 mM, what is V_K? What would you expect the resting membrane voltage to be?

6. What changes would you expect to record in the action potential if serum sodium fell to 60 mM?

7. If the resting membrane voltage suddenly changed from -70 to -80 mV, would the neuron be more or less excitable? From -70 to -60 mV?

8. Why is action potential propagation faster in myelinated nerves than in nonmyelinated nerves of the same size?

9. This time-voltage tracing shows several important portions of an action potential.

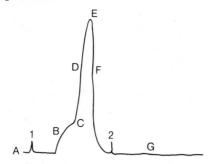

a. What is the major determinant of voltage A?
b. Following stimulus 1, what is event B?
c. What is the name we give to voltage C? What happens at this voltage?
d. What events are happening during time D?
e. What do we term voltage E?
f. What are the ionic movements in time period F?
g. Why is there no action potential following stimulus 2?

10. Succinylcholine is a widely used muscle relaxant for surgery. When it is injected, muscles show contraction "ripples" and then do not contract. The muscles will contract if stimulated directly. The resting membrane voltage at the end plate region is -40 mV. What is the mechanism of action of the paralysis?

11. Why do acetylcholinesterase inhibitors make good insecticides? What is the therapy for a human insecticide poisoning?

12. Why are end plates usually found in the center of skeletal muscles?

13. What is the source of the Ca^{2+} that activates skeletal muscle?

14. How would you expect the A band width to vary during muscle contraction? The I band width?

15. How have sensory modalities been defined for use in neurologic testing?

16. What kinds of questions would you ask a patient to elicit information on peripheral nerve function?

17. What sorts of conditions lead to rapid, extensive atrophy of muscle groups?

18. What are the major nerves of the arm?

19. How do the spinal nerves divide as they enter the spinal cord?

20. What conclusions about the location of damage can you draw if both motor and sensory function in the same region of the body are lost?

21. What is the significance of voluntary muscle weakness?

22. What is the significance of muscle weakness when it is combined with atrophy and muscle twitching?

23. Where is the lesion most likely to be if there is a total sensory loss on the back of the leg?

24. What sensory and motor deficits could be expected if the radial nerve is damaged in a fracture of the humerus?

CASE HISTORIES

1. H. S. is a 27-year-old jackhammer operator. He noticed yesterday that he had trouble spreading his right fingers to get his leather gloves on. He complains about what lousy work running a jackhammer is. He wants

to know how long he can be on workmen's compensation.

When you examine him, his interossei muscles are very weak (when he fans his fingers you can easily close them). He has no sensation in the third and fourth fingers. He has great difficulty flexing his right little finger against force.

Where in the pathway between the fingers and the spinal cord is the lesion? What is the most likely cause of the problem? What, if any, treatment should be undertaken? Should this be treated as a workmen's compensation case?

2. D. M. is a 38-year-old executive of a music conservatory. She has awoken, with increasing frequency, during the night with pains in her left hand, especially in the thumb and first two fingers. When she flexed and extended the wrist, the pains would go away. Recently the pain increased and sometimes radiates into the center of the forearm. On examination, touch as well as pain sensations are diminished in the thumb and first two fingers, particularly on the palmar surface. She cannot pull her thumb toward her nose. Her hand is slightly swollen and does not sweat.

Where in the pathway from the skin to the spinal cord is the lesion? Why doesn't the hand sweat? What is the most likely cause of the problem? Can remedial action be taken and, if so, what?

3. J. M. is a 22-year-old medical student doing his medicine rotation on your unit. You notice he seems tired about 11:00 A.M. and disappears for a nap about 1:00 P.M., much to the annoyance of everyone. After a nap or a night's sleep, he is full of vigor and always ready to run down the hall to fetch a chart. He is helping you stock a shelf at 10:30 A.M. when the sixth bottle drops out of his hands. He remarks, "I am just not as strong as I used to be." His hand grasp is indeed weak, but there is no sensory loss.

What types of problems might lead to weakness of the hand muscles? What information does the intact sensation give? What structures are intact? What diagnostic tests are indicated?

4. J. C. complains of weakness in her legs. She first noticed this yesterday in her ankles; today her knees are weak. There is possibly some weakness of her hips. She has no sensory loss or other symptoms.

What structure(s) is (are) implicated? What is the likely disease process? What is the likely course? What is the long-term prognosis?

5. (The following case has been provided by Julie DuBoise, R.N.)

Ms. S.S. is brought to the emergency room in a weakened condition. She cannot sit up and complains of generalized weakness that began approximately 12 hours earlier and has worsened throughout the day. The patient's daughter arrives soon thereafter; she has a milder version of the same symptoms. They had eaten together at a local restaurant the day before. She has double and blurred vision, difficulty in speaking and swallowing, and shortness of breath. Light hurts her eyes. An examination confirmed these sysmptoms and shows weakness in moving her respiratory muscles. She is alert and orientated, afebrile, with all sensory modalities intact but with a decrease in deep tendon reflexes.

Where is the anatomic site of her problem? What diseases act there?

6. H.R., a 38-year-old male, is in for a checkup. He has occasional periods of numbness of his hands and he "cuts" his hands more often than previously. He has decreased sensation in both hands, halfway up both forearms, and in both feet. Both hands and feet are more abraded than normal. He seems a bit weak.

What is your impression?

3

Spinal Cord

The spinal cord can be divided anatomically and functionally into two parts: *segmental* and *transmission*. Transmission to and from the brain resides in the peripheral white matter (Fig. 3-1) and will be considered later.

SEGMENTAL SPINAL CORD

The segmental function of the spinal cord lies in its central gray matter. This function is closely tied to the peripheral nervous system and has already been partially considered.

Each spinal cord segment is delimited by its pairs of spinal roots (Fig. 3-1). The segments of the spinal cord are named just as the vertebrae are, as follows: *cervical, thoracic, lumbar,* and *sacral*. As the fetus grows, the spinal cord does not grow as rapidly as does the vertebral column. As a result there is a space in the lumbar region, occupied only by spinal nerves and cerebrospinal fluid (Fig. 3-2). This is the region into which a needle is inserted for a spinal tap.

Spinal Nerves

Axons are gathered in spinal nerves as they travel between the plexus and the spinal cord. As each of the major nerves of the arm approaches the vertebral column, they join into an intricate network—the *brachial plexus* (see Fig. 2-15)—where the peripheral nerve fibers divide to form the *spinal nerves* of spinal cord segments C5 to T1. Each spinal nerve must pass through a hole, the *intervertebral foramen*, in the vertebral column to reach the spinal cord inside (Fig. 3-3).

As each spinal nerve enters this foramen, it passes through the dura. Then the spinal nerve divides into anterior and posterior roots. All the sensory fibers travel into the spinal cord in the posterior root and have their cell bodies in the posterior root ganglion (Fig. 3-1). All the motor fibers leaving the spinal cord do so in the anterior root. The *dura* is the thick, tough covering of the brain and spinal cord. Within the dural sac the central nervous system (CNS) floats in *cerebrospinal fluid*.

The individual vertebrae are held

F I G U R E 3-1
Spinal nerves enter the vertebral canal and divide into anterior (motor) and posterior (sensory) roots. The sensory axons have ther cell bodies in the posterior root ganglion and enter the posterior gray matter of the spinal cord. Motor axons have their cell bodies in the anterior gray matter. The white matter contains axons running up and down the spinal cord. (From *An Introduction to the Neurosciences*.)

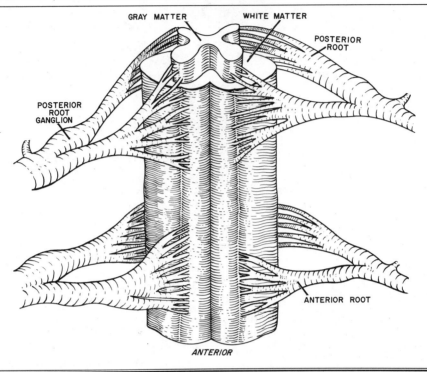

GRAY MATTER   WHITE MATTER

POSTERIOR ROOT

POSTERIOR ROOT GANGLION

ANTERIOR ROOT

ANTERIOR

F I G U R E 3-2
A sagittal magnetic resonance imaging (MRI) scan of the lumbar spine. The verterbral column, spinal cord, and spinal nerves are shown. The spinal cord ends in the junction of the thoracic and lumbar vertebrae. (MRI scan courtesy of Robert Tucker, M.D., University of Illinois College of Medicine at Peoria.)

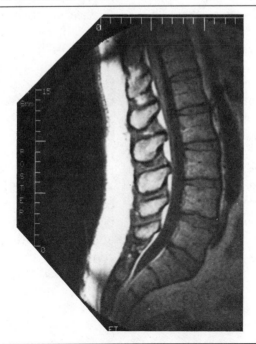

F I G U R E 3-3
(A) A three-dimensional (3D) reconstruction of a computed tomography (CT) scan of a lumbar vertebra. Only the bony structure is shown because the reconstruction ignored all the soft tissue such as the nerves. These 3D reconstructions can be done from any angle; this one was chosen to show the intervertebral foramen (*arrow*). **(B)** A midsagittal reconstructed section of the same vertebra, reconstructed as if you were inside the spinal canal, looking out. (CT scans courtesy of G. Zwicky, M.D., St. Francis Medical Center, Peoria, IL.)

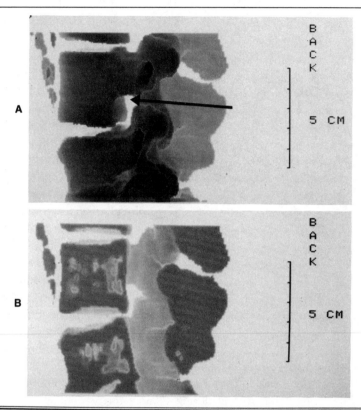

apart by the *intervertebral disks* (Fig. 3-2), which act as shock absorbers between the bony vertebrae. Each disk consists of a hard outer anulus (doughnut) and a semiliquid core. This core occasionally ruptures and protrudes from the anulus in a posterior lateral direction. If so, it puts pressure on the spinal roots or on the nerve in the intravertebral foramen or on both (Fig. 3-4). This pressure stimulates the axons in the roots, particularly in the posterior root, and gives patients the sensation of pain. The pain is referred to the area (a dermatome) where these sensory axons began. Patients often describe the pain associated with a

ruptured lumbar disk as a hot knife being dragged up the outside of their leg. Rupture most often occurs during the lifting of a heavy object or other strenuous motor activity. Continued pressure on the spinal nerve causes permanent damage to both motor and sensory nerves. The motor nerve damage may cause muscular atrophy.

C A S E   H I S T O R Y
Extruded Disk

Ms. S.B., a very active 17-year-old high school student, complained of intense pains in the lower back. During her high school career, she

F I G U R E 3-4
A ruptured intervertebral disk putting pressure on a posterior root.

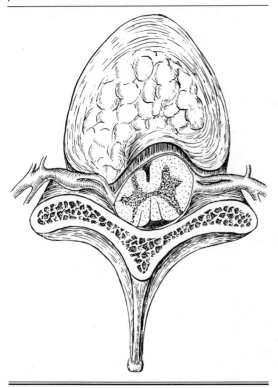

has been very active in cheerleading and in basketball. Two weeks ago, she noticed a pain in her back while doing a handspring during cheerleading. The pain disappeared. One week ago the pain returned and became so intense that any movement was painful. She lay in bed. Her chief complaint was the pain in her back. She also noted a numbness spreading down the front of her left lower leg and into her foot.

On examination, there was a significant sensory loss to pain, temperature, and light touch over the anterior surface of the left leg and foot. She was unable to tell which toe the examiner was holding, much less determine movement of that toe. Her left knee and ankle reflexes were significantly reduced. Strength was apparently intact but hard to test accurately because of the pain. On standing, which was very painful for her, she stood with her knees bent forward and her shoulders thrown back. There was considerable tenseness of the lower back muscles. On moving from side to side, which exacerbated the pain, the muscles tensed even more. The reflexes and sensation in her upper extremities were normal. She showed complete orientation to time, place, and person. The cranial nerve findings were all negative.

Shooting pains are usually caused by a hard object rubbing on a peripheral nerve, spinal nerve, or posterior root. In this case, the front of the leg is innervated by branches of the sciatic nerve or by the L4 spinal nerve or posterior root. Numbness in the same area suggests a prolonged loss of pain and temperature sensation. Indeed there was loss of all sensory modalities to the leg; this loss suggests a peripheral as opposed to a spinal cord loss.

The diminution of reflexes without loss of strength suggests a loss of the stretch receptor axons as they travel with the spinal nerve or posterior root. The pure sensory nature of the loss strongly suggests a posterior root lesion. A spinal nerve or peripheral nerve lesion usually gives both a motor and sensory loss. Much of the pain and tenseness of the lower back comes from a pain-induced reflexive contraction of the interspinus muscles. These interconnect the vertebrae and their spasm pulls the vertebrae closer together, constricts the intervertebral foramen, and causes more pain. The sudden onset of the pain strongly suggests a rupture of an intravertebral disk, as in Figure 3-4, which was confirmed on magnetic resonance imaging. The extruded disk was removed by a laminectomy, and complete recovery occurred.

Anterior Horn Cell to Muscle

Within the *anterior gray matter* of the spinal cord are large neurons called *anterior horn cells*. These cells send axons out through the anterior root to join peripheral nerves and run to muscles. When each nerve reaches its muscle, it branches and supplies a number of muscle cells.

Since each skeletal muscle cell is innervated by only one axon, it will contract only when its axon and, hence, its anterior horn cell, is activated. You will recall that all the muscle cells controlled by a single axon are called a motor unit, and they act in an identical fashion. If an anterior horn cell dies, its motor unit can no longer contract since the chain of command is broken. Polio (anterior poliomyelitis) causes paralysis by destroying many anterior horn cells.

Reflexes. Reflexes are stereotyped motor responses to well-defined stimuli. The knee-jerk response is a good example. The efferent or motor branch begins with the anterior horn cells (Fig. 3-5), which receive input from sensory neurons entering in the same or a nearby segment. These stereotyped patterns are "hard-wired" into nervous connections. One such pathway is shown in Figure 3-6. A stretch receptor in the muscle reacts

to the tap of the reflex hammer by sending off a group of action potentials in its axon, which makes a synapse on the anterior horn cell. These sensory action potentials cause the motor nerve to fire action potentials and the muscle to contract. The pathway of this reflex is fixed, but the number of muscle groups activated is not; therefore, the amount of motion is variable. If your patient locks his fingers together and pulls hard just as you strike the patellar tendon, the response will be stronger. Only motor groups in the stretched muscle react.

Stretch Reflexes. These can be easily elicited in antigravity muscles such as gastrocnemius (ankle jerk), quadriceps (knee jerk), biceps, and triceps. These reflexes persist if the spinal cord is severed higher up but are lost if the peripheral nerve is cut; they are segmental responses.

Facilitation. An input that enchances a reflex, facilitates that reflex. The example of pulling against locked fingers is an ex-

F I G U R E 3-5

A cervical spinal cord cross section showing an anterior horn cell and monosynaptic reflex pathway. (From *An Introduction to the Neurosciences.*)

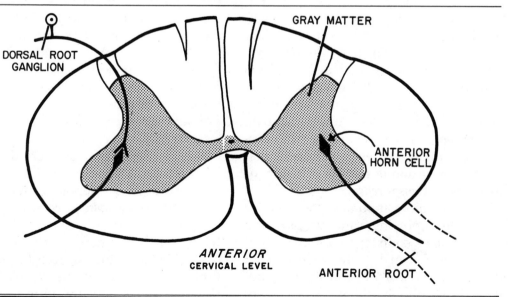

F I G U R E 3-6
A stretch reflex pathway. The axon from the stretch receptor enters the spinal cord by
the posterior root, branches, and synapses with an anterior horn cell. The motor axon
traverses the anterior root and the same peripheral nerve back to the same skeletal
muscle. (From *An Introduction to the Neurosciences.*)

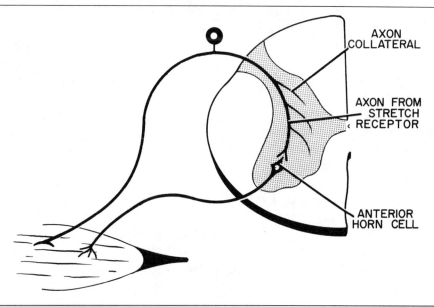

ample of facilitation. Reflexes can be much more extensive than the stretch reflexes described above; reflexive withdrawal from pain is a good example. Almost everyone has touched a hot object and jerked their hand away. This is a spinal reflex. The response is predominantly a flexor response and is graded. If two areas are burned, the response will be increased, facilitated. Pain fibers spread widely on both sides of the spinal cord for three or more segments on either side of entry. An intense pain in one foot, such as that caused by stepping on a nail, can elicit flexion in that leg and extension of the opposite leg, or the *crossed extensor reflex*.

Two or more inputs to the anterior horn cells supplying a muscle can "add up" to initiate contraction. Often each of these stimuli can be subthreshold, but their sum will be above threshold. In addition, two stimuli, either of which separately gives a small contraction, may

lead to a very large contraction if applied at the same time. We speak of this adding up of stimuli as facilitation, and it is one of the very basic mechanisms of nerve cell interaction, both in the spinal cord and in the brain.

When an electrode is placed in an anterior horn cell, a resting membrane voltage of −80 mV is recorded. Each facilitatory input depolarizes the cell and brings the resting membrane voltage toward the threshold voltage required to fire an action potential (i.e., −80 to −60mV). Nerve cells that cause facilitation release neurotransmitters that bind with receptors on an anterior horn cell and result in brief depolarizations called *excitatory post synaptic potentials* (EPSPs).

Inhibition. If one nerve cell prevents another from reacting, we call the interaction between the two nerve cells *inhibition*. We can inhibit the urge to drop a hot coffee cup during the few seconds needed to put it down. A useful example is the role inhibition plays in the movement of a joint, such as the knee. Figure 3-7 shows the knee and the two major muscle groups that control it: the quadriceps (Quad), the extensor, and bi-

ceps-semitendinosus (B-St), the flexor. When the Quad contracts, either reflexively or voluntarily, the knee is extended and the B-St is stretched. The B-St does not contract, however; the B-St stretch reflex has been inhibited by in-

F I G U R E 3-7
The cellular events (*top*) and the anatomic pathways (*bottom*) of inhibition of a stretch reflex. (See the text for further details.)

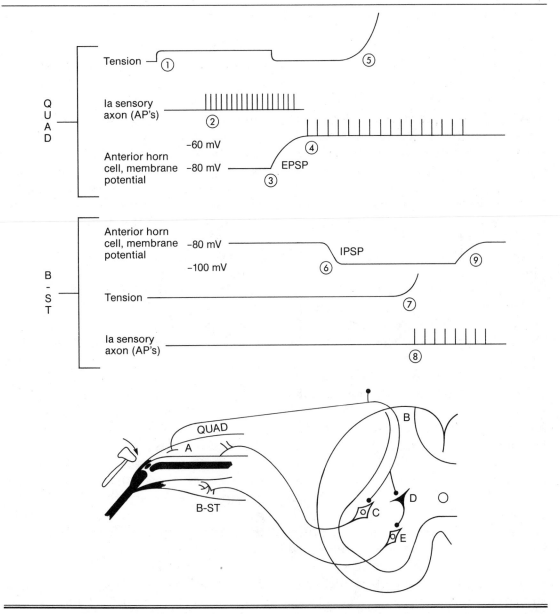

terneuron D. A similar inhibition exists at all joints between opposing muscles.

At the cellular level, inhibition is the result of neurotransmitters that cause hyperpolarization when they bind to receptors on anterior horn cells. These are a different group of neurotransmitters from those that cause facilitation. The resting membrane potential of the anterior horn cells becomes more negative (-80 to -85mV). The membrane potential is now further from threshold, and it is harder to fire an action potential. Inhibitory inputs result in *inhibitory post synaptic potentials* (IPSPs).

Let's look at Figure 3-7 step-by-step. Action begins with a brief stretch *(1)* of the Quad tendon and the resulting tension placed on the muscle. This tension activates the stretch receptors *(A)*, which begin firing action potentials *(2)*. These action potentials travel up the peripheral nerve and enter the spinal cord by the posterior horn *(B)*. As the sensory axon transverses the gray matter, it branches many times. One branch synapses on a Quad anterior horn cell *(C)*, where the released neurotransmitter causes an EPSP *(3)*. The EPSP depolarizes the anterior horn cell to threshold, and action potentials fire *(4)*. These action potentials initiate contraction in the Quad; tension is produced *(5)*, and the leg extends.

At the same time that the stretch receptor axon stimulates the Quad anterior horn cell, it activates an interneuron *(D)*, which releases a different neurotransmitter at its synaptic junction with a B-St anterior horn cell *(E)*. This second transmitter results in hyperpolarization *(6)*, an IPSP, of the B-St anterior horn cell. The IPSP is long-lasting, and the B-St anterior horn cell is still hyperpolarized when the contraction of the Quad *(5)* extends the leg and stretches the B-St *(7)*. Stretching the B-St activates stretch receptors *(8)*, which depolarize the B-St anterior horn cells *(9)*. This depolarization, whose pathway is not shown, does not cause the anterior horn cell to reach threshold because of the preceding IPSP; consequently, the B-St does not contract even though it is stretched.

Much the same pathways work when a muscle group is activated voluntarily: antagonist muscles are inhibited, and synergists are facilitated.

Stretch Receptors

Golgi Tendon Organs. These receptors are sensitive to stretch and report the tension the muscle is exerting or the static tension on the joint. The major function of these receptors is to prevent the muscle from exerting so much tension that its insertion will pull off the bone. The primary nerve ending enters the posterior root and synapses on interneurons. These in turn inhibit the anterior horn cells of the same muscle and reduce the tension. They probably play no part in stretch reflexes.

Muscle Spindles. The receptor for the stretch reflex is the muscle spindle. These dynamic receptors may well play a role in the control of muscle activity. Their structure is shown diagrammatically in Figure 3-8. Three to five small, striated muscle fibers and axon endings lie together in a spindlelike sheath, which itself lies parallel with the bulk of the muscle fibers.

Sensory fibers arising from the muscle spindle are of two types. Large, Group Ia fibers have their origin in the *annulospiral endings*, which wrap around the intrafusal fibers. These axons emit a burst of action potentials whenever the spindle is stretched to a new length and then settle down to signal a new spindle length. They "report" both rate of

F I G U R E 3-8
A muscle spindle. (From Gardner, E.: *Fundamentals of Neurology*. Philadelphia, W.B. Saunders, 1968.)

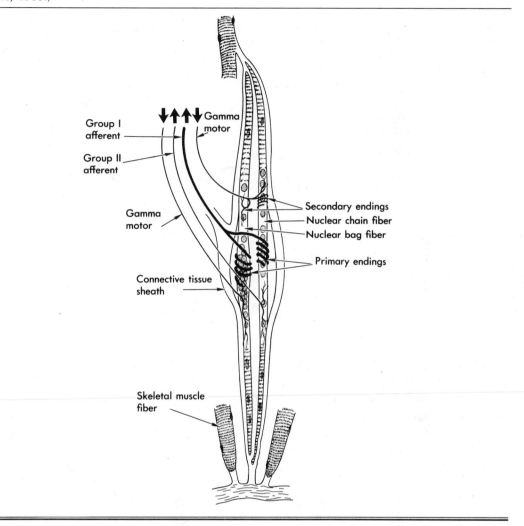

change of muscle length and the new position. These large afferent fibers from the anulospiral endings mediate the stretch reflex (Fig. 3-9). Such axons give off collaterals that rise to higher centers to signal limb movement and also branch widely within the gray matter to facilitate synergistic muscles and to inhibit antagonistic muscles.

The smaller, Group IIa afferent fibers from the *flower-spray endings* also have synaptic endings in the segments near the level of entry. These endings project to the ipsilateral cerebellum and convey information on limb position.

Gamma Motor System. The inclusion of active muscle cells within the muscle spindle makes it a fascinating and unique sensory receptor. The muscle cells inside the muscle spindles are called intrafusal fibers. They are innervated by smaller motor nerve fibers, gamma (γ) motor fibers. This contractile system is often referred to as the γ motor system. The muscle cells making up

F I G U R E 3-9
The innervation of intrafusal and extrafusal muscle fibers form α and γ anterior horn cells.

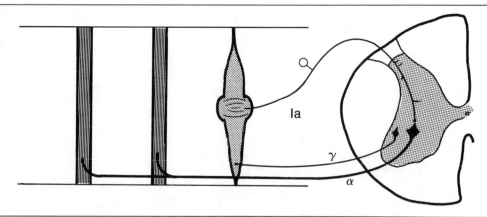

the bulk of the muscle are called extra-fusal fibers and are innervated by large α motor neurons. Both types of motor neurons arise from anterior horn cells (Fig. 3-9).

What are the functions of the intra-fusal fibers?

1. By contraction in synchrony with the extrafusal fibers, the sensitivity of the sensory fibers remains constant. Because the muscle spindle is parallel with the extrafusal fibers, maximal contraction of the extrafusal fibers would leave the muscle spindle slack. A stretch reflex cannot be obtained when the muscle spindle is slack. By contracting in synchrony with the extrafusal fibers, the muscle spindle remains taut and capable of reacting to stretch.
2. By contracting, the extrafusal fibers can increase the sensitivity of the muscle spindle. Such a mechanism may account for the "tensed-up reflexes" when walking in the dark or along a railroad rail.
3. The role of the γ system in the control of movement is under active investigation, and our current knowledge is fragmentary. The example

shown in Figure 3-10 is only partially based on fact. It uses the first finger of the left hand to uncover a tone hole in a wind instrument or depress a piano key.

The cycle begins when the contralateral frontal lobe "commands" a musical note to be produced. A burst of action potentials (1) descends in a corticospinal axon that synapses directly on the α motor neuron (A); contraction begins (2). Initial force is determined by the number of motor units activated.

At the same time, axons found in a second descending system (3)—perhaps the rubospinal tract—are activated. These in turn activate γ anterior horn cells (B). The γ anterior horn cells activate intrafusal fibers; these in turn cause the Ia fibers to react (4). The Ia fibers further stimulate the α motor neurons, and contraction is maintained after the burst of corticospinal action potentials ends.

As the muscle shortens, the muscle spindle begins to slacken and the firing rate of the Ia sensory fiber declines (5). Soon a muscle length is reached where the firing rate of the Ia

F I G U R E 3-10
A possible mechanism for controlling position. (See the text for a description.)

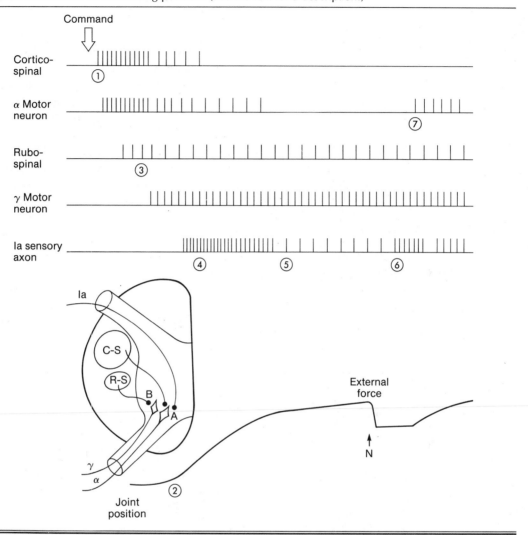

fiber is below threshold for the α motor neuron; movement ceases. Remember, however, that the γ system is still activated, and its degree of activation determines the final position.

Contrast these two systems: a direct, corticospinal, system that initiates contraction and determines the initial force, and a γ system that determines final muscle length, joint position, and final force.

After the final position of the joint has been reached, continued γ stim-ulation keeps the joint in the final position against any external force that moves the joint as at N. Immediately after movement, the Ia sensory fiber reacts with a burst of action potentials (6), which leads to increased firing of the α motor neuron (7), muscle contraction, and correction of the joint position.

Contraction might be initiated by γ activation, although with a long delay. We have no evidence that pure γ activation plays a dominant role in initiation of normal movement. It may be possible, however, to retrain a patient with damage to the corticospinal system to use other pathways and to initiate movement, perhaps by γ stimulation.

Spinal Cord Cross Sections

Cross sections from each group of the spinal cord segments—cervical, thoracic, lumbar and sacral—are shown in Figure 3-11. These cross sections vary considerably both in total size and in the relative sizes of the gray and white columns.

The white matter decreases in bulk as the distance from the brain increases. Descending motor tracts leave the white matter to influence anterior horn cells; nearly one-half do so in the cervical region to control hand and arm movements. Sensory fibers enter the cord continuously. The majority of sensory fibers enter from the limbs, so there are large increases in the white matter bulk in the cervical and lumbar regions. A cervical section contains axons running up from the thoracic, lumbar, and sacral levels as well as axons from the cervical level. The white matter columns are long, thin pyramids with their base at the foramen magnum and their tips at the sacral segments.

The situation in the spinal cord gray matter is different. Here, there are swellings and constrictions, although the gray matter is continuous. The gray mat-

F I G U R E 3-11
Cross sections of the spinal cord. Note the varying size of the gray matter. (From Goss, C.F.: *Gray's Anatomy*. Philadelphia, Lea & Febiger, 1986.)

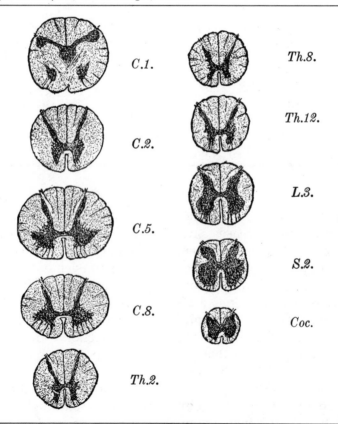

ter sends, receives, and integrates information to and from a particular segment of the body. Its bulk at any particular segment depends on the precision of movement and the subtlety of sensory response of that segment. The precise movement of the hand is reflected in small motor units. Hence there are many anterior horn cells and large anterior horns in the cervical segments that innervate the hand. The subtlety of sensory response in the arm and leg are subtended by a large number of sensory axons, which have rich synapses in the gray matter of cervical and lumbar segments. Consequently, the posterior horns of these segments are large, while the posterior horns of the thoracic and sacral segments are relatively small.

Segments can be recognized by the relative amounts of white and gray matter. Cervical sections have roughly equal amounts of white and gray matter and an oval shape. Lumbar segments have almost as much gray and less white. The thoracic segments are mostly white matter with long, thin posterior horns. Sacral segments are small and are composed of mostly gray matter.

TRANSMISSION IN THE SPINAL CORD

Sensory Systems

Pain and Temperature. Sensory fibers from the pain and temperature receptors enter the spinal cord, synapse extensively, and cross the midline within three segments of entry (Fig. 3-12). Sensory fibers rise in the opposite side of the spinal cord and ultimately reach the contralateral postcentral gyrus. For example, pain fibers from the right foot rise in the left lateral spinal cord by way of the left *spinothalamic tract*.

Pain fibers add to the medial and posterior side of the tract so that the spinothalamic tract is laminated. Fibers

FIGURE 3-12
The transmission pathway for pain and temperature sensation. The synaptic chain in the posterior root is very important in the control of pain perception.

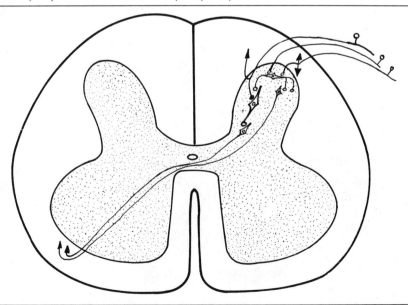

from the sacral dermatomes are found anterior and lateral, while the fibers from the cervical dermatomes are located in a more medial and posterior position. Pressure from outside the cord, as from a tumor, is more likely to block transmission in fibers from the sacral area last.

The rich synaptic connections that pain and temperature fibers make in the posterior horn are very important in altering the perception of pain. The relation between the physical or organic injury and the perceived pain is highly variable; a distance runner can "ignore" considerable muscle and joint pain until the end of the race; similarly, women in labor can often divert their attention away from pain. The perception of pain is also altered when the area surrounding a wound is rubbed or licked, thereby stimulating large-diameter nerve fibers.

Most of the gating of pain transmission by large-diameter peripheral fibers and by descending fibers occurs in the posterior horn. It is of great significance that receptors for the endorphins (the body's own narcotics) are located in the posterior horn. Synaptic transmission in this area is being studied intensely because of the possibility of blocking pain transmission from only part of the body and of avoiding the side effects of systemic therapy.

When pain fibers from a region have been lost, whether temporarily or permanently, higher sensory centers in the upper brain stem respond by referring the sensation of numbness to the region. The crossed leg "falling asleep" is an example.

Position and Vibration. Axons from vibration receptors enter the spinal cord and rise on the same side (Fig. 3-13). These fibers do not synapse or cross the neuroaxis until they reach the brain stem. The nerve fibers stimulated by a vibrating tuning fork placed on the left thumb rise in the left side of the spinal cord. The tracts, called the *posterior columns,* are laminated. The entering fibers add to the lateral surface of the column; in the cervical region the fibers from the

F I G U R E 3-13
The transmission pathway for vibration and position sensation.

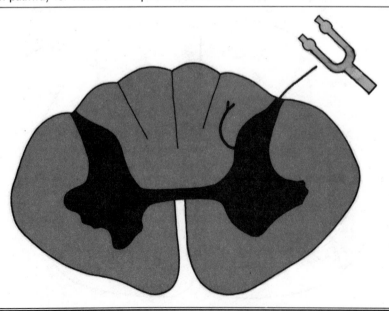

legs are medial and the fibers from the arms are lateral.

Touch. Axons carrying information about touch and pressure sensation enter the spinal cord, usually synapse, and rise in both the posterior and anterior columns on both sides. Discrete spinal cord lesions rarely cause loss of touch sensation. Hence loss of touch sensation to a region is a sign of a peripheral lesion and is usually accompanied by loss of other sensory modalities and lower motor neuron signs.

The position of the joints is transmitted to the cerebellum by the *spinocerebellar tracts,* which lie in the lateral columns. Unconscious position sense from the right leg travels on the right side of the cord to the right cerebellar hemisphere.

Motor Systems

Voluntary Motor Control. The frontal lobe commands for muscle activation are transmitted in the spinal cord on the same side as the muscle activated by the *corticospinal tracts.* The nerve fibers leave the corticospinal tract and synapse on interneurons whose axons, in turn, synapse on anterior horn cells (Fig. 3-14). This tract has its origin in the frontal lobe on the contralateral side, crosses the neuroaxis in the brain stem, and then runs ipsilaterally in the spinal cord.

The corticospinal tract also influences the reflexive response of the toes to a mildly painful stimulus made to the lateral sole of the foot. In normal adults, the toes curl up (flex) (Fig. 3-15). In infants and in adults with damage to the corticospinal tract, the large toe extends and the other toes spread. This response, called *Babinski's reflex* or *sign,* is usually the first evidence of damage, such as pressure from a tumor, to the corticospinal tract.

Muscle Tone. The degree of resistance of muscle to passive stretch, such as movement by an examiner, is described as muscle tone. If an arm is very floppy, as in an unconscious patient, or if a muscle

F I G U R E 3-14
The transmission pathway for voluntary motor control.

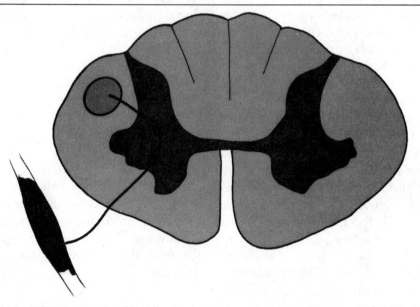

F I G U R E 3-15
Responses to stroking the sole of the foot. **(A)** The normal adult response. **(B)** The pathologic adult response; the Babinski's sign.

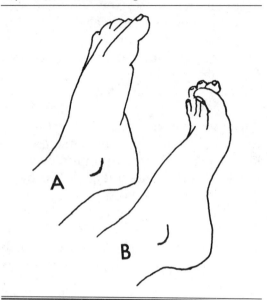

or a limb is without motor nerves, the tone is described as *flaccid*. If the limb is very stiff and hard to move, it is described as *spastic*. In general, when the spastic limb is moved very slowly, there is little resistance. If the joint is moved rapidly, there is a brief, free interval followed by rapidly increasing resistance to stretch. Loss of function of the corticospinal tract is largely responsible for spasticity. Ischemia, pressure, or severing of this tract produces spasticity.

When an examiner moves a spastic leg, the resistance to stretch quickly mounts until there is a sudden release of tension. This sequence of increasing resistance to passive stretch followed abruptly by relaxation is called the *clasp-knife reflex* and is thought to be mediated by the Golgi tendon organs. When the reflexes of both the extensor and flexor of the ankle are active, a rapid push of the toes toward the patient will result in a sustained back and forth motion, called *clonus*, another sign of corticospinal tract damage.

Voluntary Weakness. Loss of muscle strength is a frequent presenting complaint and is one of the cornerstones of neurologic diagnosis. If the anterior horn, spinal root, or spinal nerve is the site of the damage, we speak of a *lower motor neuron lesion*. We would expect a weak, flaccid muscle without a reflex (areflexic) that shows gross atrophy and frequent twitching (fasciculations). Lesions of the neuromuscular junction and muscle give similar losses. An *upper motor neuron lesion* results from damage to the corticospinal tract from its origin in the frontal lobe to the exit of its fibers from the lateral column. We expect a spastic paralysis, hyperreflexia, and a Babinski's sign but only minimal disuse atrophy. Clonus may be present.

In addition to the corticospinal tract, there is descending motor influence from the brain stem. This travels in a number of tracts in the anterior and lateral columns: the vestibulospinal, the rubrospinal, and the reticulospinal tracts (see Fig. 3-17). We will discuss them further in later chapters. Our overall knowledge of these tracts is limited, but they generally enhance extensor reflexes in the legs and flexor reflexes in the arms. These tracts are often lumped together and called the extrapyramidal system.

LESIONS

Hemisection

Consider the lesion shown in Figure 3-16, which destroyed the left half of the first and second lumbar segments. It is often referred to as the Brown-Séquard syndrome. The examiner would expect to find the following deficits in such cases:

1. A lower motor neuron lesion to the

F I G U R E 3-16
A hemisection of the lumbar cord.

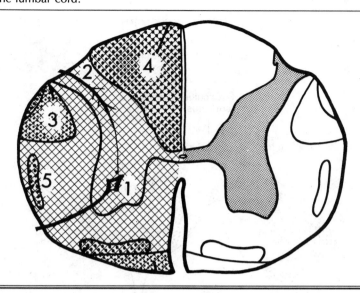

hip and thigh muscles controlled by these segments would be present. There would be a flaccid paralysis of the left hip; it would move easily in the examiner's hands. The left knee jerk would be diminished or absent.

2. A total sensory loss (touch, pain and temperature, and position sense) due to destruction of the entire posterior root would be present over the left anterior thigh.

3. An upper motor neuron lesion caused by the cutting of the corticospinal tract would be present. All the muscles supplied by segments below the lesion would show a spastic paralysis and hyperreflexia. The muscles of the left lower leg would be affected, and there would be an exaggerated left ankle jerk. A left Babinski's sign would be present.

4. The cutting of the ascending fibers of the posterior columns would block all vibration and position sense from the same side of the body from the hip down the left leg.

5. Interruption of the lateral spinotha-

lamic tract would block all pain and temperature fibers which have reached the tract at L2. Because pain and temperature fibers take up to three segments to cross the neuroaxis, the loss begins in the L5 dermatome (see Figs. 2-13 and 2-14), the back of the right leg and buttocks.

Disease Types

Intervertebral disk rupture (extrusion) has already been discussed. Trauma frequently causes partial or complete cord transection, particularly in the cervical region. The edema accompanying trauma often causes extensive dysfunction that clears in four to six weeks.

Tumors. Space-occupying neoplasms of the spinal cord lie primarily outside the spinal cord proper and produce symptoms by pressing on spinal roots or the spinal cord itself. Pain, referred to the dermatome innervated by the spinal root, is a common symptom. Compression of the spinal cord blocks transmis-

F I G U R E 3-17
The major tracts of the spinal cord.

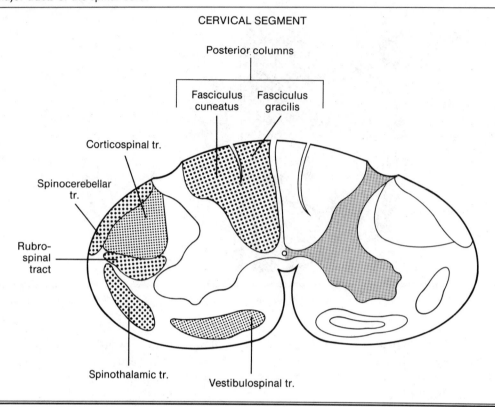

CERVICAL SEGMENT

Posterior columns

Fasciculus cuneatus   Fasciculus gracilis

Corticospinal tr.

Spinocerebellar tr.

Rubro-spinal tract

Spinothalamic tr.

Vestibulospinal tr.

sion of impulses and leads to sensory and motor deficits; clumsiness is a common symptom. Tumors can usually be diagnosed by a history of increasing, unremitting symptoms often over a period of several months or years. Magnetic resonance imaging is very useful in diagnosing spinal cord lesions, is not invasive, and does not expose the patient to radiation. Surgical removal of the tumor is usually successful. If unrecognized, these tumors will transect the spinal cord.

C A S E   H I S T O R Y
Spinal Cord Compression

Hank J. had been a first-string end on his high school football team for 2 years and was start-

ing spring practice. His coach noticed a clumsiness in the drills for foot control, particularly of the left foot. The trainer found no relevant history but did find a markedly decreased ability to feel vibration at both ankles and knees. Both ankle jerks were brisk, with the left more active than the right. There was a Babinski's response on the left. Touch sensation was unchanged. Hank was referred to a neurosurgeon who confirmed these findings and also found a band of greatly decreased touch and pain sensation on the right side of the trunk just above the umbilicus.

All these signs pointed to an extrinsic tumor compressing the spinal cord in the thoracic region. After the tumor was removed, there was a brief, total paralysis of the legs followed by complete recovery; Hank was able to play the next season.

This case illustrates the primary principle of neurologic diagnosis: finding a locus where a single lesion can cause all the signs and symptoms. Hank J.'s lesion was unlikely to be in the peripheral nerves to the legs because touch sensation was intact. The motor nerves are probably unaffected because the reflexes are brisk rather than absent. The loss of vibratory sensation in both legs, but not the arms, suggested both posterior columns were damaged somewhere above the lumbar level but below the cervical level.

The motor findings (brisk reflexes and positive Babinski's sign) were upper motor neuron findings. The major motor tract, the corticospinal tract, was also damaged but not destroyed somewhere between the precentral gyrus and the lower spinal cord. The damage might have been to the precentral gyrus or in the spinal cord below the cervical level (the arms are unaffected). The missing piece of information found by the neurosurgeon was a sign that related to a segmental function; in this case, the tumor destroyed all sensory modalities on the right side of the trunk. These modalities enter the cord by way of two or three right posterior roots. This is an example of a level lesion; all the problems were caused by disease at a single locus.

Spinal Shock. After a spinal cord injury, particularly a transection, a flaccid, areflexic paralysis develops below the lesion. This is known as spinal shock. If the transection is complete, voluntary muscle control and sensation will never be recovered. Often the transection is not complete but tissue swelling or vascular insufficiency cause a functional transection that will clear in 1 to 3 months when some motor or sensory tracts begin to function. During the early weeks the areflexia is total, and the lack of bladder and bowel emptying is of particular concern. If careful bladder emptying is not instituted, kidney infection and death will follow.

If the transection is complete, in 2 to 6 weeks flexion relexes begin to return to the segments below the transection, often starting with Babinski's response. Months later any small stimulus may lead to a mass flexion. After a year or so, extensor spasm often replaces flexor spasms. Bladder emptying returns, sometimes with voluntary control, although the pathway is unknown. While direct treatment is not possible, physical and occupational therapy can help these patients lead useful lives.

Systems Diseases. For various reasons, some disease processes attack only certain systems or cell types and leave others intact. Hence the disease process can be found wherever the afflicted system is found in the nervous system. *Poliomyelitis* is a viral infection of the anterior horn cells and causes classic lower motor neuron symptoms. *Amyotrophic lateral sclerosis* (ALS) attacks both anterior horn cells and corticospinal fibers, giving a combination of upper and lower motor neuron signs. It is primarily a disease of middle years and is more common in males. The cause is unknown, there is no specific treatment, and death usually occurs 3 to 5 years after symptoms appear.

A lack of vitamin B12 causes degeneration primarily of the posterior columns and corticospinal tracts; this degeneration is known as *combined system disease*. Its progression can be halted and some symptoms reversed by weekly injections of vitamin B12. Other disease processes can spread thoughout the neuroaxis. *Multiple sclerosis* causes patchy demyelination and a loss of function of both white and gray matter in the spinal cord. The case history in Chapter 4 is illustrative. *Metastatic carcinoma* causes both single and multiple lesions with symptoms arising by compression of nervous tissue.

Bladder Reflexes

Stretch receptors in the detrusor muscle of the bladder and pain receptors of the bladder mucosa send fibers into S2-4 spinal cord segments to make contact with anterior horn cells. Motor fibers run back to the detrusor and external sphincter muscles. As the bladder fills with urine, the wall stretches and impulses enter the posterior horn and activate motor neurons. We learn to suppress this reflex consciously until some socially convenient time. The infant with an unmyelinated corticospinal tract or the adult with high bilateral damage to the corticospinal tract has no pathway to suppress the reflex. Whenever the bladder fills, it empties completely by reflex action. A patient in spinal shock has temporarily lost the reflex. Consequently, the bladder must be catheterized to prevent overstretching the wall and destroying the receptors so that when reflex action returns to the sacral cord, the bladder will empty reflexively. Patients with destruction of the sacral cord will never regain the emptying reflex and will need intermittent catheterization.

POST-TEST

1. How are the vertebral and spinal cord segments classified?

2. Where do sensory nerves enter the spinal cord?

3. When do the nerves carrying pain and temperature sensation cross the neuroaxis?

4. How do you define a spinal reflex?

5. Define the conditions of the affected muscles when there is slow damage to the descending motor tracts.

6. What is the pathway for voluntary motor control by way of the corticospinal tract, beginning in the precentral gyrus?

7. What is the significance of unilateral Babinski's response in an adult?

8. What conclusions can you draw from a muscle that is flaccid and gives occasional spontaneous twitches?

9. What deficit would cause a loss of position and vibratory sense below the umbilicus?

10. What conclusions can you draw when the only deficits are loss of pain and temperature from the umbilicus to the costal margin on both right and left sides?

11. Define upper and lower motor neuron lesions and the signs and symptoms each causes.

12. Where is the lesion if a muscle is strong and has normal tone and bulk but is areflexic?

CASE HISTORIES

Identify each structure or tract involved. Try to locate the level of the lesion and describe the pathology.

1. Mr. A.J. has noticed gradual weakness of his left arm over the last few months; now he cannot pick up his bowling ball with it. When questioned, he reports that his right leg is often numb. Examination reveals decreased strength, decreased muscle bulk, and hyporeflexia in the left arm. There is decreased strength and hyperreflexia in the left leg. There is a positive Babinski's reflex in both feet. Pain and temperature sensation is decreased in the right leg and on the right side of the body up to the level of the nipple. Often he is not aware of the examiner's pinprick.

2. Ms. C.M., a 42-year-old housewife, has had a pain in her left arm and shoulder for the past year or so. She cannot pinpoint the time of onset other than "about the time my youngest started school." The pain varies; sometimes it has a dull quality in the left shoulder, while at other times it radiates down the left arm to the elbow. Occasionally the pain is so intense that she takes a painkiller to get to sleep. On examination there is a decrease in pain and temperature sensation in the left arm from the shoulder to the elbow and a decreased vibratory sensation at the elbow and acromion. Light touch is decreased in the same general area. There is a decrease in pain and temperature sensation on the right side below the shoulder. The muscles of the left upper arm are weak in comparison with those of the right and seem to be smaller. All other examination is negative.

3. Ms. J.R. has noted a gradual loss of control of her right foot, which has made driving her car more difficult. The right ankle and knee jerks are hyperactive, both toes are upgoing, and right ankle flexion and extension are weak. Pinprick, touch, and position and vibratory sense are intact, but two-point discrimination is diminished. She cannot identify numbers drawn on her right foot.

4. Ms. J.C. is a 36-year-old secretary who for a year or so has noticed an increased clumsiness both in walking and in typing. On examination she shows decreased vibratory sense in her right and left legs, right arm, and on most vertebral spines. Position sense at the right toes is markedly decreased, as it is in the right hand. Other sensory modalities are intact.

She shows a positive Babinski's reflex on the left and has questionably increased elbow jerks.

5. Mr. J.Q. is a much-tattooed ex-sailor who is now a garage mechanic. He has a gash in his left forefinger. After putting in six stitches you ask about his general health. He replies, "Nothing much wrong, just some tingling in the legs." On examination you find a marked decrease in position and vibratory sense in both legs and decreased knee and ankle jerks. Strength and muscle bulk in the legs are unimpared. There is a mild decrease in pain and light touch sensibility in no specific pattern over parts of both legs.

6. J.C. is a 17-year-old basketball player. Her coach has noted clumsiness in J.C.'s left leg. She does remember occasional "pins and needles" of her left leg whenever she crossed her legs. On examination you find decreased strength in the left ankle and a decreased ankle jerk. Pain, touch and position, and vibration are diminished just below the left knee.

7. Mr. A.H. is a 56-year-old foundry worker who was in excellent health until 3 years ago when he recalls becoming more tired than usual after a day's work. He had to take it easy on the weekends to "rest up" for the next week's work. This tiredness gradually increased so much that he had to be transferred within his company to a lighter job. Now he can walk up stairs only if he stops at the landing to rest. On examination the muscles of the arms and legs appear very small for a man of his build. Occasional twitching is noted in the finger and scapula muscles. The deep tendon reflexes of the arms and legs are very brisk and symmetrical. There is no sensory deficit.

LESION DIAGRAMS

SAMPLE PAGE
YOU SHOULD WORK UP EACH OF THE LESION DIAGRAMS IN THIS MANNER:

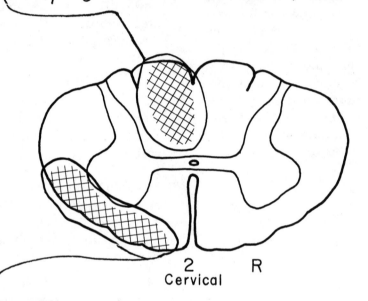

Location: Lt. posterior column
Major Tract: posterior column
Modality interrupted: position & vibratory sense
Body region affected: Lt. ankle & knee

2 R
Cervical

Location: Lateral-anterior white column
Major Tract: L. Lateral spino-thalamic
Modality interrupted: pain & temperature
Body region affected: Rt. side, below shoulder

LESION DIAGRAMS

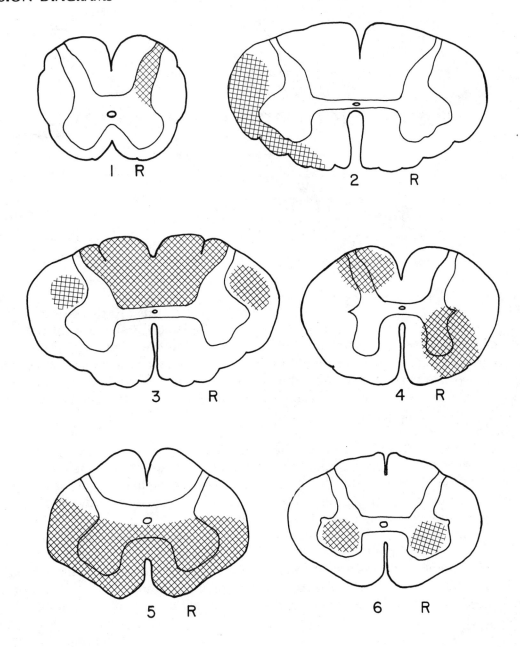

4

Brain Stem and Cerebellum

BRAIN STEM

The neuroaxis enters the skull through the foramen magnum to form the brain stem, which has many features in common with the spinal cord but adds some new features to distinguish it as part of the brain.

All sensory tracts rising up from the spinal cord continue on through the brain stem on their way to the cerebrum. The main motor tract, the *corticospinal tract*, runs down the entire length of the brain stem. Of the 12 cranial nerves, 11 run to or from the brain stem; they carry motor and sensory information for the head and neck. The cerebrum sends commands to the cranial nerve nuclei by the *corticobulbar tract*. In addition, the brain stem controls and regulates a number of general body functions such as cardiovascular and respiratory function and our state of wakefulness.

The major subdivisions of the brain stem (Fig. 4-1) are the medulla, pons, midbrain, and diencephalon. These regions have discrete functions, and each contains groupings of cell bodies (called nuclei) and bundles of axons (called

tracts). In contrast to those of the spinal cord, the tracts and nuclei of the brain stem are intermingled.

The *medulla* is a direct continuation of the spinal cord and contains fiber tracts that are continuations of those in the spinal cord. It also contains groups of motor and sensory nuclei for its segments, which are the throat, neck, and mouth. In addition, the medulla exhibits reflex activities involved in the control of the respiratory and cardiovascular systems.

The *pons* contains cranial nerve nuclei associated with sensory input from and motor outflow to the face. The large bulge of the brain stem so typical of the pons is made up of fibers coursing down from the cerebrum, synapsing and running up into the cerebellum.

The *midbrain* contains the major motor nuclei controlling eye movement. It contains a huge pair of tracts—the corticobulbar and corticospinal—carrying signals down from the cerebral hemispheres. The midbrain also contains all the ascending sensory tracts.

The *diencephalon* is the highest portion of the brain stem. The major sensory tracts that have traversed the spinal

F I G U R E 4-1
The subdivisions of the brain stem.

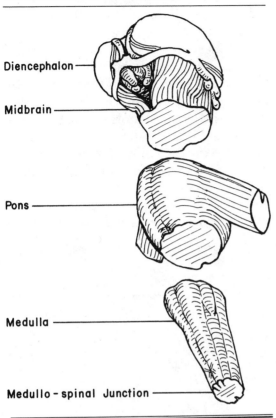

Diencephalon

Midbrain

Pons

Medulla

Medullo - spinal Junction

cord and brain stem synapse here, as do the visual and auditory pathways.

Posterior Fossa

This rigid subdivision of the cranial cavity is occupied by the brain stem and cerebellum (Fig. 4-2). The roof of the cavity is a thick, parchmentlike circular sheet whose periphery attaches to the skull. This is the *tentorium*, which lies over the cerebellum. Anteriorly there is a semicircular opening, the *tentorial notch* or *incisura*, which fits snugly around the midbrain to define the upper boundary of the posterior fossa. The *foramen magnum*, a large hole in the skull at the bottom of the posterior fossa, lets the brain stem in.

At both the foramen magnum and the tentorium, the nervous tissue fits the holes fairly closely. The brain stem and cerebellum also fit fairly snugly into the cavity of the posterior fossa. Trouble occurs when there is an expanding, space-occupying lesion in the fossa, either inside or outside the brain itself. The growth or swelling quickly takes up the small leftover space and then begins to compress the remaining brain material.

F I G U R E 4-2
The posterior fossa contains the brain stem and cerebellum. The arrows show the level of the tentorium. (MRI scan courtesy of Gerald Palagallo, M.D.)

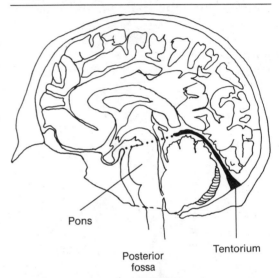

Pons

Posterior fossa

Tentorium

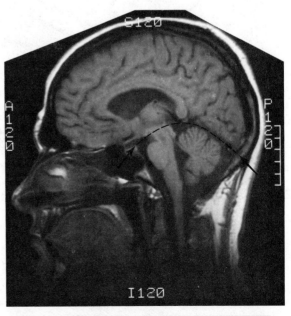

As in the spinal cord, compressed nervous tissue functions poorly, if at all. In an attempt to create more room, *herniation* occurs: brain tissue moves toward and through the foramen magnum, the tentorial notch, or both. An expanding lesion above the tentorium can force the cerebrum down through the tentorium and cause pressure on the midbrain.

Figure 4-3 is a view of the base (bottom) of the skull from above, with the tentorium shown on the right side. The midbrain is seen emerging through the tentorial notch. Cranial nerve III emerges from the midbrain and runs under the tentorium to a special groove in the base of the skull. The cavity shown on the right side is occupied by the temporal lobe, which floats above the third cranial nerve.

The left side of the diagram shows the medial surface of the temporal lobe being forced down and into the tentorial notch; the arrow denotes pressure. This movement of the temporal lobe puts pressure on the third cranial nerve and causes it to cease functioning. The first function to be lost is pupil constriction. As a result, the pupil is dilated and does not constrict when a light is shined on

F I G U R E 4-3
Herniation of the temporal lobe onto cranial nerve III.

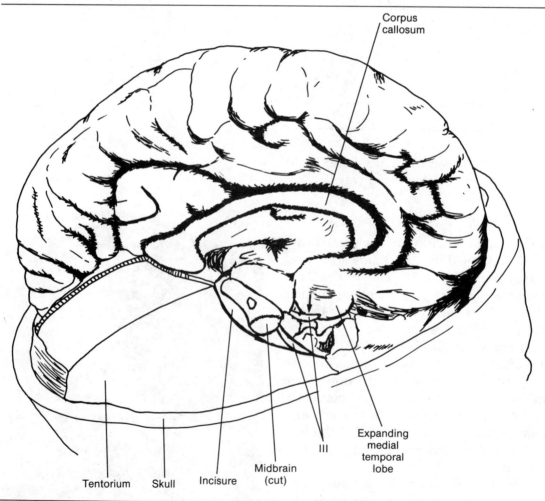

the eye. An increase in pressure forces the medial surface even further into the tentorial notch and can sever the midbrain. Pupils not reacting to light, particularly in an unconscious or partly conscious patient, is a life-threatening situation that needs immediate neurosugical consultation.

Increased pressure in the posterior fossa causes changes in the retina that can be seen with an ophthalmoscope. The normal pulsation in the optic veins decreases or is absent with increasing intercranial pressure. The optic vein empties into the posterior fossa, and increasing pressure there is reflected back into the eye in a damming-up effect. The optic nerve is normally sunken below the surrounding retina. Increasing pressure in the posterior fossa causes *papilledema,* elevation of the disk and blurring of the margins. Axonal transport of enzymes and fluid from the cell bodies in the retina to the synaptic terminals in the diencephalon is interrupted. The distal end of the nerve swells, like a bulging garden hose.

CEREBELLUM

The cerebellum is the largest structure in the posterior fossa. The specific functions of parts of the cerebellum are hard to define precisely at the present state of our knowledge; only gross functions can be tested. I will speculate further on its function in Chapter 6.

The crebellum makes three major connections on each side of the neuroaxis (Fig. 4-4). The *inferior cerebellar peduncles* receive the spinocerebellar tracts and input from the vestibular nuclei of the medulla, which bring information on

F I G U R E 4-4
The cerebellar peduncles.

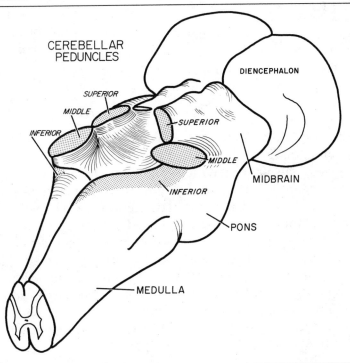

the position of the body. The inferior cerebellar peduncle also carries signals back to the vestibular nuclei and influences posture by the vestibulospinal tract.

The *middle cerebellar peduncles* receive signals from the cerebrum by way of tracts that synapse in the pons, turn, and run into the cerebellum. These are command signals, asking for directions, for example, to get the right finger to the nose. The cortex and deep nuclei of the cerebellum compare the two signals—one indicating where the limbs are and the other indicating where they are commanded to be—and produce a difference signal. This difference signal leaves the cerebellum by the *superior cerebellar peduncle* and travels up the neuroaxis to the higher brain stem, particularly to the thalamus of the diencephalon. (The middle and superior peduncles will be seen later in Figs. 4-10 and 4-11.)

Tests of Cerebellar Function

These tests assume that the individual muscles have reasonable strength for the task required, and that the sensory tracts from the spinal cord to the cerebrum are intact. A normal person should be able to reach out and touch the examiner's finger and then move his hand smoothly and quickly back to touch his own nose. The patient with cerebellar pathology shows coarse side-to-side movements during the motion. The same is true of running the heel up the shin. These tests should be made in both right and left arms and legs. The patient with a cerebellar lesion has great difficulty standing with feet together and has a staggering, ataxic gait with feet well apart, as does a person who has consumed too much alcohol.

MEDULLA

Tracts

The vitally important sensory tracts of the spinal cord, which have been gathering information from all of the body below the neck, continue into the medulla. The descending motor command fibers flow through the medulla on their way to the anterior horn cells of the spinal cord. In the low medulla the major descending motor tract, the *corticospinal tract*, crosses the neuroaxis. Signals from the left precentral gyrus cross to the right side, where they continue in the spinal cord.

The ascending *posterior columns* cross the neuroaxis in the midmedulla. Nerve fibers carrying position and vibration sensation enter the spinal cord, go directly into the posterior columns of the same side, and continue on the same side throughout the spinal cord. The *spinothalamic tract* contains pain and temperature fibers from the contralateral side of the body and continues in an anterior and lateral position. In the high medulla, all the major tracts are contralateral.

Cranial Nerves

The medulla is the origin of a number of cranial nerves (Fig. 4-5). These include the *hypoglossal*, or cranial nerve XII, which sends motor fibers to the muscles of the tongue. The voluntary pathway is tested by asking the patient to stick out his tongue. Any deviation of the point of the tongue from straight ahead points to the side of the lesion. Destruction of the motor nucleus in the medulla or the nerve pathway is signaled by atrophy and twitching of the tongue in addition to paralysis.

F I G U R E 4-5
The cranial nerves of the medulla.

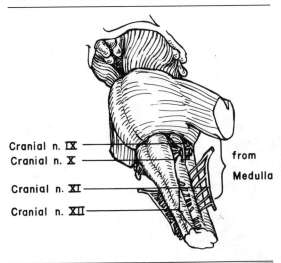

Cranial n. IX
Cranial n. X
Cranial n. XI
Cranial n. XII

from
Medulla

The *spinal accessory,* or cranial nerve XI, sends motor fibers to the sternomastoid and trapezius muscles. Function is tested by asking the patient to turn his head and shrug his shoulders against the resistance of the examiner's hand. Remember that the right sternomastoid muscle turns the head to the left.

Cranial nerves IX and X, the *glossopharyngeal* and *vagus,* are considered together since they both arise from the same region of the medulla and exit the brain stem and skull in the same region. They often get into trouble together. They both innervate the back of the mouth and throat. The sensory input from the back of the mouth and top of the throat is responsible for much of our ability to taste, swallow, and gag.

The muscles of this region, especially the *soft palate,* are important in swallowing. The function of these fibers, both sensory and motor, is tested by stroking the tonsils with a tongue depressor. The patient gags, frequently at the sight of the tongue depressor. It is important to observe if the uvula that hangs down from the soft palate rises in the midline.

If the soft palate cannot rise, liquid is regurgitated through the nose. When liquid is forced backward by the tongue rising, it escapes around the soft palate into the nasal cavity instead of being forced down the throat and esophagus. The vagus innervates the muscles of the larynx; paralysis leads to a hoarse voice. The vagus also sends fibers to most of the abdominal organs.

Brain Functions

The medulla controls both the *cardiovascular* and *pulmonary* systems. The pulmonary system is controlled on a breath-by-breath basis by medullary respiratory centers. The receptors that control breathing are CO_2 receptors in the medulla itself. The primary O_2 receptors are in the neck at the branching of the common carotid. The O_2 receptors act as a fail-safe system and do not usually control respiration. Hypoxia of the medulla does, however, activate the respiratory center. The cardiovascular system is controlled by several groups of cells that act to regulate a constant blood pressure through control of both heart rate and peripheral blood flow.

The center that coordinates swallowing, nausea, and vomiting is located in the medulla. Nausea or vomiting or both for longer than 8 to 12 hours should make you think about pressure in the posterior fossa as a possible cause. Syrup of ipecac specifically activates the vomiting center and is useful in ridding the body of many poisons. Identify the probable poison first! Caustic and petroleum products should be pumped out.

A Cross Section (Figs. 4-6 and 4-7)

A horizontal section through the lower third of the medulla is shown in Figure 4-6A, and an outline drawing of the ma-

F I G U R E 4-6
(A) A myelin stained cross section of the human medulla. (Courtesy of S. Jacobson, Ph.D., from *An Introduction to the Neurosciences*.) **(B)** An outline drawing of this section of the midmedulla. Tracts are stippled and labeled on the right; nuclei on the left. (Anterior structures, such as the corticospinal tract, are oriented upwards, to conform with the convention of magnetic resonance imaging (MRI) scans. Many texts use the opposite convention.)

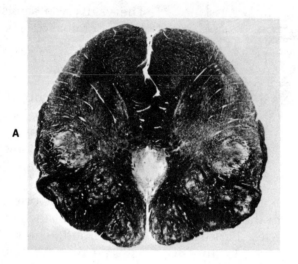

A

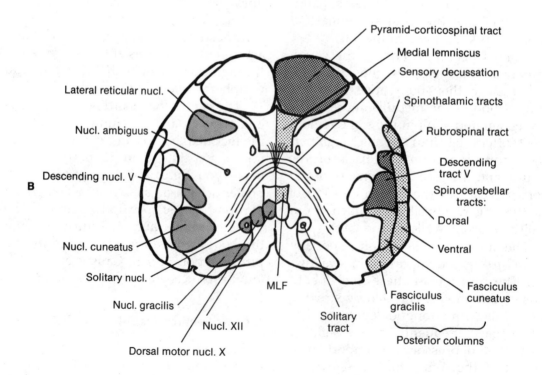

B

F I G U R E 4-7
(A) An axial magnetic resonance imaging (MRI) scan of the medulla and surrounding cerebellum. (Courtesy of Gerald Palagallo, M.D.) **(B)** A labeled outline drawing.

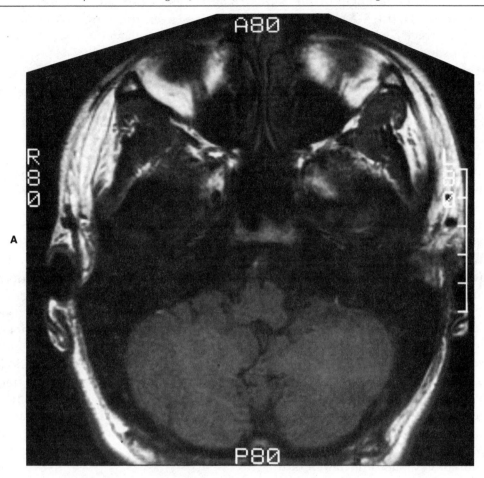

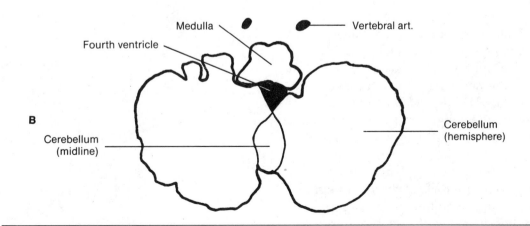

jor structures appears in Figure 4-6B. An MRI scan of approximately the same level but at a different angle of the section is shown in Figure 4-7A.

The fiber tracts, which are symmetrical, are labeled on the right side of Figure 4-6. The pyramid contains the *corticospinal tract*, which controls voluntary motion. Here the corticospinal tract is contralateral because the crossing, or decussation, occurs lower in the brain stem at the medulla-spinal cord junction (see Fig. 4-1). The *spinothalamic tract* (carrying pain and temperature sensation) retains its anterior-lateral position as in the spinal cord. Remember that these axons synapsed and crossed the neuroaxis as they entered the cord. The *posterior columns* (carrying position and vibration sensation) end at this level in large synaptic regions called the nuclei cuneatus and gracilis. Axons leaving these nuclei cross the neuroaxis to form the *medial lemniscus*, which rises to the thalamus as a contralateral tract. The *spinocerebellar tracts* retain their lateral position and are ipsilateral.

The *descending tract* and *nucleus of the fifth cranial nerve* run throughout the medulla and convey pain and temperature sensations from the ipsilateral face. These fibers enter as the trigeminal nerve (V) in the pons, descend in the tract, synapse in the nucleus, cross the neuroaxis, and rise to the thalamus with the medial lemniscus (see Fig. 4-9).

This section of the medulla (Fig. 4-6) contains three motor nuclei, long cylinders of motor cell bodies, which run along the neuroaxis through most of the medulla. The *hypoglossal nucleus* (XII) controls the tongue muscles. The *dorsal motor nucleus of the vagus* (X) supplies preganglionic parasympathetic innervation to the salivary glands, heart, and the gut. The *nucleus ambiguus* integrates swallowing, vomiting, and gagging and supplies fibers to the glossopharyngeal

(IX) nerve. The *nucleus solitarius* gathers fibers carrying taste sensation from cranial nerves IX and VII, which carry these impulses from the tongue and oral cavity to the medulla.

PONS

Cranial Nerves (Fig. 4-8)

Cranial nerve VIII or the *vestibuloacoustic nerve* receives the sensory fibers from the organs of hearing and balance. Neural deafness in one ear is almost always associated with nerve VIII damage. Once inside the brain stem, the fibers from each ear disperse widely as they rise to the transverse temporal gyrus of the temporal lobe. Each temporal lobe receives about one-half the fibers of each ear.

Total auditory function is tested by holding a vibrating tuning fork on the mastoid process. If the patient can ·"hear" it buzzing, the end organ and nerve VIII are intact. Patients who cannot hear the tuning fork buzzing when

F I G U R E 4-8
The cranial nerves of the pons.

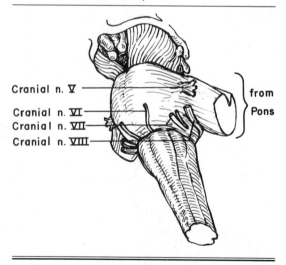

Cranial n. V

Cranial n. VI
Cranial n. VII
Cranial n. VIII

from Pons

it is placed on the mastoid process have *neural deafness* caused either by end-organ disease or nerve VIII damage. The tuning fork should be held at the mastoid until the patient can no longer feel it. Then the vibrating tuning fork should be placed next to the external ear. If the patient can hear it, the conduction system for sound through the ear canal and the bones of the middle ear is intact. If the patient cannot hear it, he or she is suffering from *conduction deafness,* which can usually be remedied by a hearing aid or by surgery.

The vestibular division of the eighth cranial nerve has its origin in the semicircular canals. It conveys information on the body's position in space and is particularly sensitive to rapid changes in position. This information influences posture and eye movement.

Cranial nerve VII, or the *facial nerve,* supplies motor nerves to the muscles of facial expression. Wrinkling of the forehead by looking up, closing the eyes, and pulling back the corners of the mouth are the most often tested functions. Voluntary movements are controlled by nerve fibers coming down to the pons from the cerebrum in the corticobulbar tract. The right precentral gyrus controls the left side of the face.

Paralysis of the muscles innervated by one cranial nerve VII can occur as the result of either a loss of the descending command fibers (an upper motor neuron lesion) or because of the loss of the VII nerve itself (a lower motor neuron lesion).

A loss of the descending control fibers leaves the patient able to wrinkle the forehead bilaterally, but he cannot close his eye tightly. The paralyzed muscles can still participate in facial movements such as grimacing or blinking. The *corneal reflex* functions; a wisp of cotton touched to the eyeball elicits a vigorous blink response.

By contrast, a lower motor neuron lesion either to nucleus of VII or nerve VII causes complete paralysis. The corner of the mouth droops, and frequently saliva drools from it. The eye-blink reflex is lost; it is important to protect the cornea from abrasion and drying out. If the entire nerve is damaged, salivation is reduced and taste from the front of the tongue is absent. *Bell's palsy* is caused by sudden swelling around the motor nerve, with subsequent loss of motor function. It often clears in one to six months and frequently leaves little deficit.

Cranial nerve VI, or the *abducens nerve,* arises in the pons and, on leaving the brain stem, makes a long run through the posterior fossa before entering the skull to innervate the lateral rectus muscle of the eye. The long run through cerebrospinal fluid makes nerve VI especially sensitive to loss of function in patients with increased intercranial pressure. We will consider its function later when eye movement is discussed.

Cranial nerve V, or the *trigeminal nerve,* contains the main sensory nerve from the face and mouth. Pain and temperature fibers are tested by pinprick at several places on both sides of the face. Light touch should also be tested. The corneal reflex is tested by having the patient look in the opposite direction and touching the cornea with a wisp of cotton pulled to a fine point.

The motor branch of cranial nerve V innervates the muscles of jaw movement, which consists of both closure and side-to-side motion. The muscles are tested by palpation when the jaw is clenched. The stretch reflexes of the jaw are tested by lightly tapping the chin. This motor nerve exhibits both upper and lower motor neuron signs.

Cranial nerve V enters in the high pons (Fig. 4-9), and the fibers immediately divide. All fibers mediating touch

A posterior view of the brain stem showing the major functional divisions of the
trigeminal nerve (cranial nerve V).

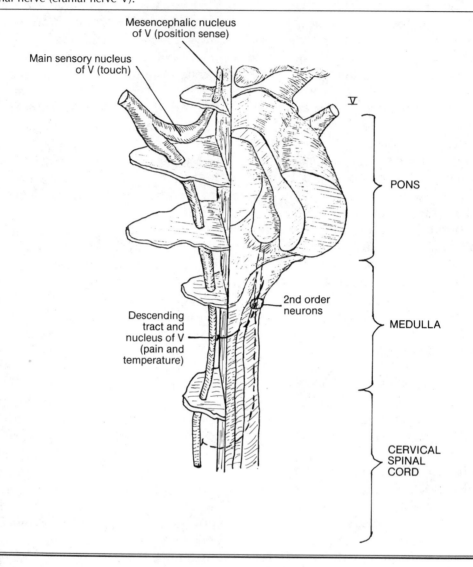

sensation enter the main sensory nucleus at the level of entry. All fibers mediating position sense enter the mesencephalic nucleus just above the level of
entry.

The fibers mediating sense of pain
and temperature descend through the
pons, medulla, and high cervical levels
(Fig. 4-9). As they descend, they leave
the descending tract of cranial nerve V
and enter descending nucleus. This nucleus is homologous to the posterior

horn of the spinal cord; indeed, the cervical portion of the descending nucleus
is continuous with the posterior horn.
Axons rise from the descending nucleus
of V, cross the neuroaxis, and rise—together with the medial lemniscus—to
the contralateral thalamus. Control of
transmission of pain information presumably occurs across the synaptic connections in the descending nucleus. Corticobulbar fibers entering the descending
nucleus may carry inhibitory impulses.

Trigeminal neuralgia is a very painful affliction of the fifth cranial nerve. Patients have frequent attacks of lancing pains in part of one side of the face. Drug therapy and surgery are often helpful.

A Cross Section

Sections of the upper pons (Figs. 4-10 and 4-11) look very different from the medulla. A major cause of this difference is the presence of major fiber tracts running to and from the cerebellum. The *middle cerebellar peduncle* is formed by fibers running first from the frontal lobe to the interlaminar nuclei of the pons, then synapsing and running up to the cerebellum. These fibers bring the command signals from the cerebrum to the cerebellum.

The sections seen in Figures 4-10 and 4-11 do not show the inferior cerebellar peduncle that lies at the pontomedullary junction at the entry of the seventh and eighth cranial nerves (see Fig. 4-8). The spinocerebellar tracts enter the cerebellum here, carrying information on where the limbs are in space. The cerebellum can then compare where the limbs are and where the cerebrum desires them to be. This "difference" signal leaves the cerebellum by the superior cerebellar peduncles, posterior to the fourth ventricle. The superior cerebellar penduncles cross the midline and run to the diencephalon and the group of motor nuclei nearby.

The trigeminal nerve enters the pons, and its nuclei are shown in Figure 4-10. Remember that the pain and temperature fibers from the face run down through the medulla before crossing and rising on the opposite side (see Fig. 4-9). The superior olivary nucleus is one of several nuclear groups in the projection of acoustic fibers to the temporal lobe.

Tracts

The great fiber tracts, with which you should be becoming familiar, continue in the pons. The spinothalamic tract (carrying contralateral pain and temperature sensation) and the medial lemniscus (carrying contralateral position and vibration sensation) continue through the pons in a posterior and lateral position. The corticospinal tract is diffuse, having entered the pons along with the corticopontine fibers. It regathers in the lower pons to form the pyramid of the medulla. The pons contains three important tracts that interconnect the brainstem nuclei. The median longitudinal fasciculus (MLF) interconnects the nuclei subserving eye movement and will be discussed later. The central tegmental tract connects the reticular formation of the medulla with that of the midbrain. The dorsal longitudinal fasciculus (DLF) carries fibers of the autonomic nervous system.

CASE HISTORY
Acoustic Neuronoma

Mrs. H.O., a 49-year-old woman, has had a hearing problem in her right ear for 6 to 7 years. At first, she had a ringing in the right ear. Five years ago, a salesman fit her with a hearing aid. About 2 years ago, she noted an unsteadiness in walking and a numbness on the right side of her face. A few months ago she began to experience episodes of unexplained nausea with occasional vomiting. Her son noted that her smile was lopsided. Now she is losing weight because of the nausea and vomiting. She has a decrease in pain and temperature sensation over the whole right side of the face with a depressed, but still-present, corneal reflex. She can neither hear nor feel a tuning fork in the right ear. The right facial muscles are weak. Walking is on a broad base, and she refuses to stand with her feet together because she is afraid of falling.

F I G U R E 4-10

(A) A myelin-stained cross section of the pons. (Courtesy of S. Jacobson, Ph.D. from *An Introduction to the Neurosciences*.) **(B)** An outline drawing of a cross section of the pons. Tracts are stippled and labeled on the right; nuclei on the left.

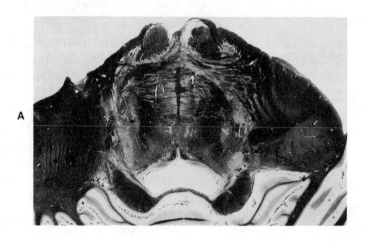

A

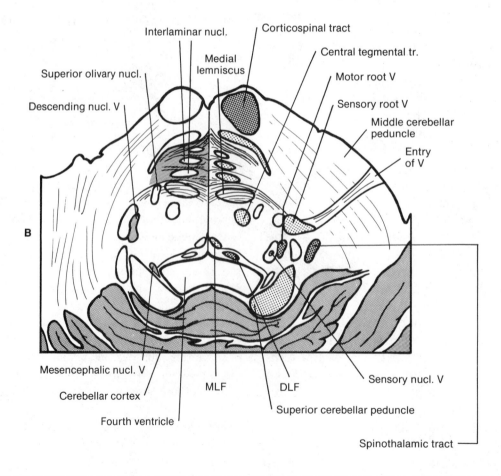

B

Interlaminar nucl.

Corticospinal tract

Medial lemniscus

Central tegmental tr.

Superior olivary nucl.

Motor root V

Descending nucl. V

Sensory root V

Middle cerebellar peduncle

Entry of V

Mesencephalic nucl. V

Sensory nucl. V

Cerebellar cortex

MLF

DLF

Superior cerebellar peduncle

Fourth ventricle

Spinothalamic tract

F I G U R E 4-11
(A) An axial magnetic resonance imaging (MRI) scan of the pons at the entry of cranial nerve V. (Courtesy of Gerald Palagallo, M.D.) **(B)** A labeled outline drawing.

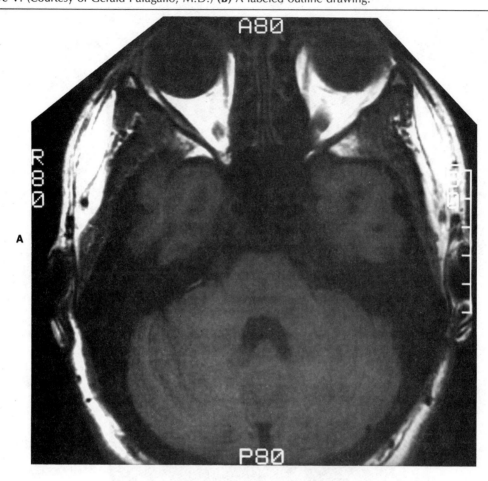

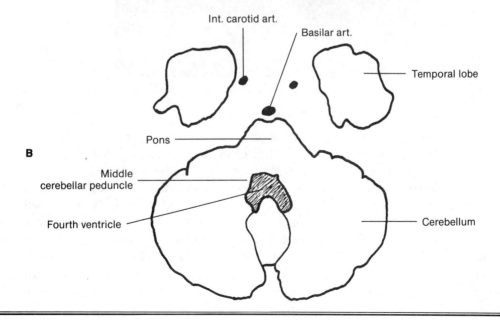

F I G U R E 4-12
A magnetic resonance imaging (MRI) scan of an acoustic neuroma. **A,** axial section; **B,**
coronal section. (Courtesy of Gerald Palagallo, M.D.)

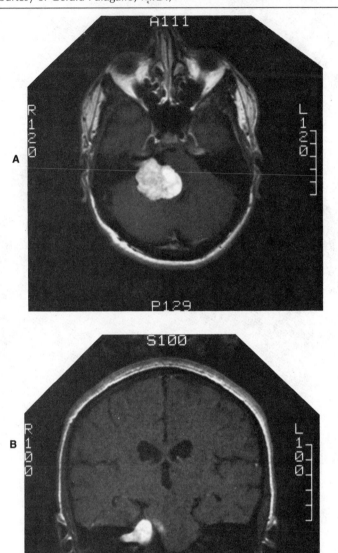

The early involvement of right cranial nerve VIII with later involvement of right VII suggests a problem at or near their common exit from the brain stem (see Fig. 4-8), just anterior to the inferior and middle cerebellar peduncles (see Fig. 4-4). The slow but insidious onset strongly suggests a tumor; the nausea and vomiting suggest the tumor is occupying space in the posterior fossa. The cranial nerve V neuropathy, decreased pain and temperature sensation in the right side of the face and decreased corneal reflex, may result either from extension of the tumor to the entry of cranial nerve V or from pressure on the descending tract of nerve V (see Fig. 4-9). The MRI scans shown in Figure 4-12 were obtained. It shows a large mass in the angle between the pons, medulla, and cerebellum.

During right suboccipital craniotomy, a tumor was removed. It was an acoustic neuroma, rising from cranial nerve VIII, surrounding nerve VII and pressing on nerve V. Two weeks after surgery the right corneal reflex was brisk, and pain and temperature sensation were returning to the right face. The patient had a deficit in the right facial muscles that never cleared. If this lesion had been diagnosed several years earlier, surgery with a stereomicroscope might well have spared nerve VII.

MIDBRAIN

Eye Movements

The six extraocular muscles in each eye move the eyeballs. The four most important of the muscles are shown in Figure 4-13. The *lateral rectus* pulls the pupil away from the nose; it is innervated by

F I G U R E 4-14
The median longitudinal fasciculus (MLF) connecting cranial nerves VI and III nuclei.

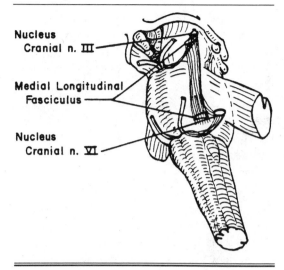

cranial nerve VI or the *abducens nerve,* which arises in the low pons and has a long run outside the brain stem before entering the skull at the level of the midbrain (Fig. 4-14).

The other muscles shown are innervated by cranial nerve III, the *oculomotor,* which arises in the midbrain and leaves the posterior fossa before running to the orbit (see Fig. 4-3). Elevation of the eyelid is also controlled by cranial nerve III. There are two other sets of eye muscles not shown, the inferior oblique, innervated by cranial nerve III, and the superior oblique, innervated by nerve IV. These muscles play a secondary role in eye movement and will not be considered further. The ocular muscles are tested by having the patient follow a flashlight or your finger with his eyes only.

In addition to the ability to move each eyeball, the muscles and their control system must be able to move both eyes together so that the image of the object falls in analogous places on both retinas. This is known as *conjugate gaze.* If conjugate gaze does not occur, the pa-

F I G U R E 4-13
The major extraocular eye muscles and their innervation.

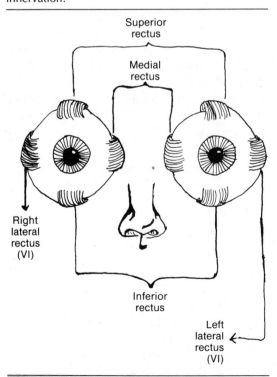

tient complains of seeing double, or *diplopia*.

The most complex coordination is in horizontal movement of the eye, which is controlled by the lateral and medial rectus muscles. The VI motor nucleus controlling the lateral rectus is some distance from the III nucleus controlling the medial rectus (Fig. 4-14), yet they must work in unison. The two are connected by a fiber tract, the MLF. Think for a moment about the eye movements involved in following a car crossing your field of view from right to left. At first the right eye is pulled fully to the right, toward the temples (temporally), by the lateral rectus. The left eye is also fully right, toward the nose (nasally), pulled there by the medial rectus. As the car moves, so do the eyeballs. This keeps the image of the car in exactly analogous positions on both retinas so that only one car is "seen." As the car passes the point in front of your nose, the horizontal eye muscles take on opposite functions. The left eye moves out by means of the lateral rectus, and the right eye moves toward the nose by its medial rectus.

Command signals for voluntary horizontal gaze "look to the right" begin in the contralateral frontal lobe and descend with the corticobulbar fibers. Command signals for involuntary visual tracking arise in the occipital lobe and also descend by corticobulbar fibers. Both command signals end in two groups of cells, near the VI nuclei, the *horizontal gaze centers* (Fig. 4-15). A command, "look to the right," descends to the right lateral gaze center; this activates the right VI nucleus and causes contraction of the right lateral rectus. The right eye turns out. At the same time, signals from the horizontal gaze center enter the left MLF to activate the left III nucleus and nerve; the left medial rectus contracts, and the left eye turns in.

Whenever the two eyes are not looking at exactly the same place, you have the sensation of seeing two versions of what you know, or suspect, to be one object. This is called diplopia, and it has three common causes.

In *nerve VI palsy*, one or both eyes cannot turn outward, either on command or in following an object. Frequently the affected eye looks inward at rest; the strong medial rectus is unopposed. Nerve VI has a long intracranial course around the bulge of the pons (see Fig. 4-14) before it reaches the level of nerve III and exits the cranial cavity to the orbit. Increasing intracranial pressure or an expanding mass in the posterior fossa is the most common cause of a nonfunctioning nerve VI.

An MLF lesion prevents commands of the horizontal gaze center from reaching the III nucleus. Consequently, one or both eyes do not move inward on horizontal gaze. The most common cause of this lesion is multiple sclerosis.

A nerve III or nucleus lesion results in one or both eyes being unable to turn in, either on horizontal gaze or convergence. An aneurysm, or bulging, of the internal carotid artery and a stroke in the midbrain are common causes.

Occasionally when the eye is pulled to extreme positions, it begins a to-and-fro motion called *nystagmus*. This is an important physical finding and indicates pathology in the posterior fossa.

Pupil Size

The iris contains two sets of muscles that vary pupillary size (Fig. 4-16) to suit light conditions. In bright light the pupil is small, and in dim light it is large. The constrictor muscles are activated when excess light enters either eye. The midbrain controls pupil size. Nerve impulses reach the two sets of muscles by widely different anatomic and pharmacologic paths. The constrictor muscles

FIGURE 4-15
A schematic diagram of the control of conjugate horizontal gaze.

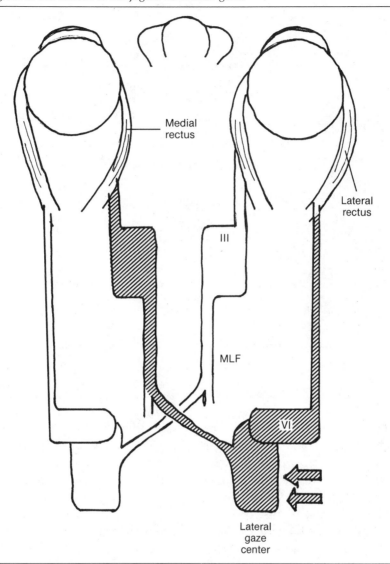

Medial
rectus

Lateral
rectus

III

MLF

VI

Lateral
gaze
center

are innervated by a branch of cranial nerve III with acetylcholine as the transmitter. The dilator muscles, on the other hand, receive innervation from the sympathetic nervous system by way of the spinal cord and sympathetic nerves in the neck with norepinephrine as the transmitter.

If cranial nerve III is interrupted or pressed on, the dilator muscles are un-opposed. This creates large pupils that do not respond to light. The most likely cause of fixed, dilated pupils is pressure on nerve III as it leaves the posterior fossa just below the tentorium (see Fig. 4-3). An expanding lesion above the tentorium is the most likely cause. The pupils may be dilated on either or both sides. Fixed, dilated pupils always indicate an emergency situation, and a neu-

F I G U R E 4-16
Nervous pathways of pupillary control.

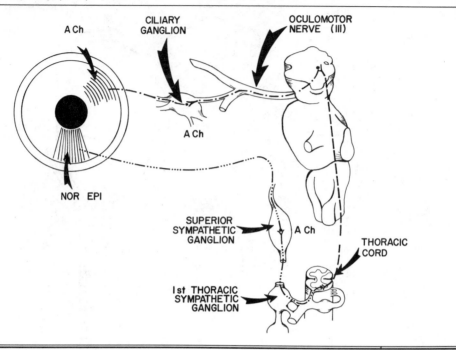

rosurgical consultation should be sought at once.

If the sympathetic supply from the neck is impaired, the constrictor muscle is unopposed and the pupil is very small. The same side of the face is usually flushed and dry because of loss of the sympathetic supply. This triad of findings is known as Horner's syndrome. Many street drugs block sympathetic transmission and result in small pupils.

C A S E   H I S T O R Y
Multiple Sclerosis

A 32-year-old mother of four, Mrs. E.B., was well until 4 years ago when she awoke one morning with tingling pains in her right leg and trunk. When she pinched her right thigh, she could hardly feel it. The tingling and the loss of pain sensation lasted for about a week and went away. Eight months later, the tingling returned together with weakness of the left hand.

The weakness went away quickly, but the tingling and partial anesthesia remained for the last 3 months of her third pregnancy. Normal feeling returned with delivery.

Two years later when being examined during her fourth pregnancy, her right side up to the breast was insensitive to pinprick, and the grip of her left hand was weak. Shortly afterwards she had diplopia for a week or so. Pinprick sensation on the right side has never returned, and the left hand has become weaker until it is now nonfunctional. The diplopia came and went but gradually became worse. At this examination, neither eye can follow a horizontally moving object across the nose; the eyes can, however, follow the examiner's finger in toward the nose. The tongue shows marked atrophy on the right and shows fasciculation on the left. On gag stimulation, the uvula rises weakly and to the right. The patient has trouble swallowing all food and regurgitates water through her nose.

This patient clearly has several sites of neurologic disease: The first site is at a low cervical level, producing the left-hand weakness and interrupting the left pain pathway carrying pain information from the right side. The second site is at the MLF in the pons, causing problems with eye movement. The last site is in the low medulla, destroying the IX, X, and XII nuclei.

The pattern of remission, exacerbation, and slow spread to discrete patches of the neuroaxis is characteristic of multiple sclerosis. Multiple sclerosis usually begins in the third decade and is more common in women. The severity and duration of the first few attacks can be reduced by corticosteroid or corticotropin (ACTH). The disease has an autoimmune component, and some cases respond to immunosuppression therapy. Palliative measures for the symptoms are of great help to the patient. Most patients lead productive, although limited, lives for many years.

Brain Functions

The *midbrain reticular formation,* or periaqueductal gray, plays an important role in controlling the state of wakefulness. It is also involved in the sudden waking up caused by noise associated with a dangerous situation. Most long-term comas can be traced to this region.

A Cross Section

Sections of the high midbrain are shown in Figures 4-17 and 4-18. The massive *cerebral peduncles* carry almost all outflow from the cerebrum. The center third of each side carries the contralateral *corticospinal tract,* and the inner third the *corticobulbar tract.* Corticobulbar tracts carry commands from the cerebrum to the brain stem. Almost one-third of the precentral gyrus relates to movement of the face and tongue. Other large portions of the frontal lobe coordinate facial and eye movements. The descending motor fibers from these areas form the corticobulbar tract and travel along with the corticospinal tract through the internal

capsule and the basis peduncle (Fig. 4-18). Just below the cerebral peduncle, the corticobulbar fibers separate and course posteriorly to innervate the cranial nerve nuclei, often bilaterally; that is, fibers in the right corticobulbar tract innervate both right and left nuclei.

The spinothalamic tract and medial lemniscus are close together, laterally and posteriorly. They enter the thalamus of the diencephalon just a little higher in the neuroaxis.

The *red nucleus* and *substantia nigra* are two major structures in the motor system. Their function will be discussed in Chapter 6.

The *oculomotor nucleus (III) and nerve* lie in this section as do the nuclei controlling pupil size. The MLF lies lateral to the nucleus of III and carries fibers important in coodinating eye movement.

DIENCEPHALON

Visual Pathways

The visual receptors are in the retina. From the retina the *optic* or cranial nerve II runs across the base of the cerebrum to the diencephalon. After a synapse in the lateral geniculate body of the diencephalon, the visual pathway continues to the medial occipital lobe (Fig. 4-19).

The visual field is divided in two by a vertical line running through the nose. Figure 4-19 shows visual fields for each eye; there is really one visual field seen by both eyes, but they are shown in this way for convenience. The visual fields are named for the patient's right and left hands. The left visual field projects onto the nasal retina of the left eye and the temporal retina of the right eye. At the chiasm, the fibers from the left nasal retina cross the midline and run with the

F I G U R E 4-17
(A) A myelin-stained cross section of the midbrain. **(B)** A diagram of this cross section
of the midbrain. The tracts are stippled and labeled on the right; the nuclei on the left.

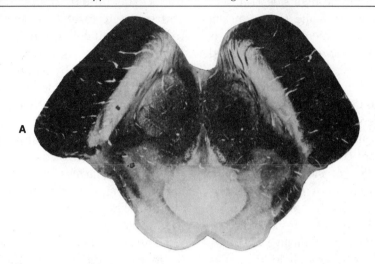

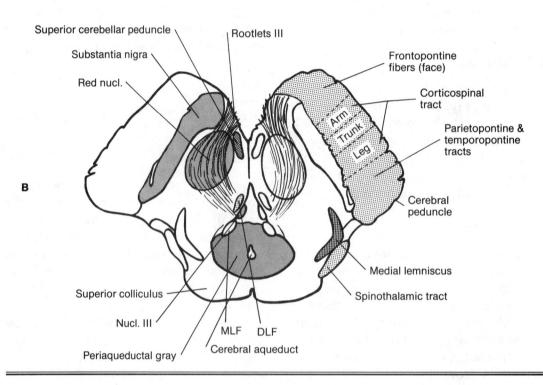

fibers from the right temporal retina to the lateral geniculate body of the thalamus. By this crossing, all the information from the left visual field is brought together in the right lateral geniculate body and subsequently the right calcarine cortex. The fibers of the right nasal retina likewise cross in the chiasm. Thus, the visual pathway repeats the usual pattern of sensory systems, where the right side is represented in the left cerebrum.

F I G U R E 4-18

(A) An axial magnetic resonance imaging (MRI) scan of the midbrain. (Courtesy of Gerald Palagallo, M.D.) **(B)** A labeled outline drawing.

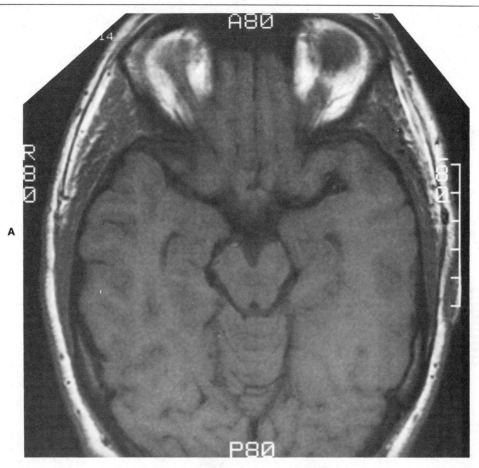

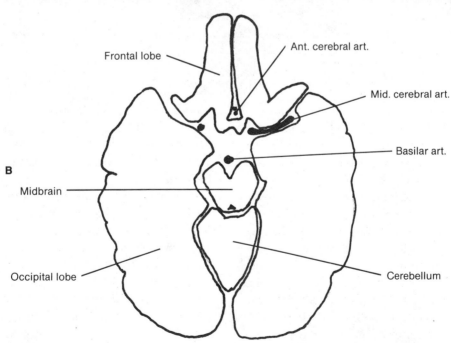

F I G U R E 4-19
The visual pathway and common lesions causing visual field deficits.

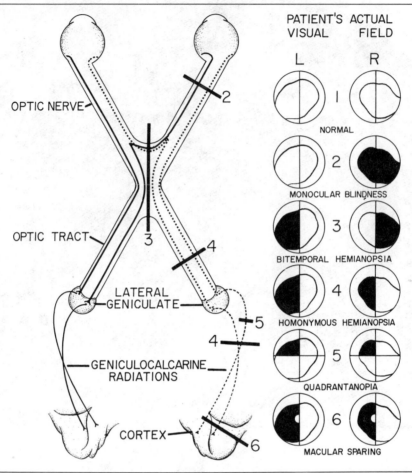

There are a number of common lesions of the visual tract with which you should be familiar. Visual fields are tested by asking the patient to cover one eye and look directly at the examiner's nose while the examiner stands about four feet away. A white-headed pin in the examiner's hand is slowly brought into the visual field until the patient sees it. The pin should be brought in from the top, the bottom, the horizontal, and the two midpoints. The visual field can be tested quantitatively with a perimeter, an instrument that does these ma-neuvers and marks them on a card. The records in Figure 4-19 are examples. The normal visual field is not symmetrical because the nose blocks vision toward the center.

If the retina or the optic nerve is destroyed (2 in Fig. 4-19), there is no sight in that eye, and *monocular blindness* results. When the lesion is in the chiasm, the fibers from both nasal retinas (temporal visual fields) are affected; the result is *bitemporal hemianopsia* (3 in Fig. 4-19). A frequent cause of this lesion is a pituitary tumor expanding upward (Fig.

F I G U R E 4-20
A coronal magnetic-resonance imaging scan (MRI) of a pituitary mass stretching the optic chiasm. Just above the mass is the third ventricle with the two thalami on either side. (MRI scan courtesy of Gerald Palagallo, M.D.)

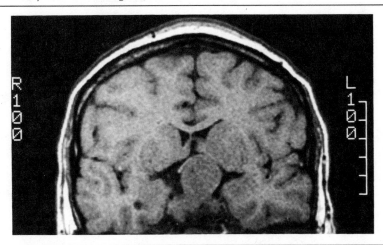

4-20). The lowermost fibers are interrupted first so that the superior temporal fields are impaired first. Complete cuts of the optic tract, the lateral geniculate body, or the geniculocalcarine radiation result in blindness in one visual field or *homonymous hemianopsia* (4 in Fig. 4-19).

Thalamus

A paired structure, this large collection of nuclei and synapses is the most superior part of the brain stem. They lie on either side of the third ventricle, deeply buried in the cerebrum (see Fig. 5-11). The thalamus serves as a relay station for all sensory fibers entering the cerebrum. Pain can be felt at the level of the thalamus but cannot be accurately localized. The sensation of peripheral numbness has its origin in the thalamus.

Large portions of the thalamus communicate to and from cortical areas and receive input from deep motor nuclei (such as the red nucleus and substantia nigra) and the cerebellum. We will discuss these in Chapter 6.

Hypothalamus

This group of nuclei lies at the base of the brain, beneath the thalamus, just above the optic chiasm and the pituitary. In the hypothalamus are the primary centers for the control of body temperature, appetite, and water excretion. The hypothalamus is also the center for many very primitive emotional reactions, such as a "fighting mad" rage and the fight-or-flight impluse. The hypothalamus exerts control over the pituitary and links the nervous and endocrine systems.

CRANIAL NERVES

Nerve	Ask About	Test
I. Olfactory	Funny smells, no smell	Both nostrils with cigarettes, other common smells
II. Optic	Can read telephone directory, see all colors, flashing lights, blackouts	Acuity: newspaper, visual fields; examine retina
III. Oculomotor	Double vision	Eye movement up, down, in
IV. Trochlear		Eye movement, convergent
VI. Abducens		Eye movement, out
V. Trigeminal	Pain in face	Pinprick in face, corneal reflex, jaw muscles
VII. Facial	Trouble moving facial muscles	Facial symmetry, smile, wrinkle forehead
VIII. Vestibular, acoustic	Balance, hearing	Hear watch; hear, feel tuning fork
IX. Glossopharyngeal	Trouble swallowing	Gag
X. Vagus	Hoarseness	Vocal cord movement
XI. Accessory		Trapezius, sternomastoid strength
XII. Hypoglossal		Stick out tongue

POST-TEST

1. What is the location in the brain stem of the pain and temperature fibers from the right leg (right or left side, anterior, posterior, or lateral)? Does it change as the tract ascends?

2. What is the location in the brain stem of the corticospinal tract to the right leg (right or left side, anterior, posterior, or lateral)? Does the location change as the tract descends?

3. Which cranial nerves subserve conjugate horizontal gaze? Where are they located? How are they connected?

4. What nerves subserve the gag reflex? What is the significance of the uvula deviating to the right on gag?

5. What is the significance of fasciculation of the tongue?

6. A patient has the sudden loss of voluntary movement on the left side of the face. What structure(s) could be affected?

7. What are the major divisions of the trigeminal (cranial V) nerve? What are the major diseases or malfunctions of this nerve?

8. Why is lateral rectus palsy an early sign of increased intracranial pressure?

9. What are some of the brainlike functions of the brain stem?

10. What structures occupy the posterior fossa?

LESION DIAGRAMS: BRAIN STEM

What loss(es) of functions will each of the following lesions (hatched areas) create? What type of disease process might be involved?

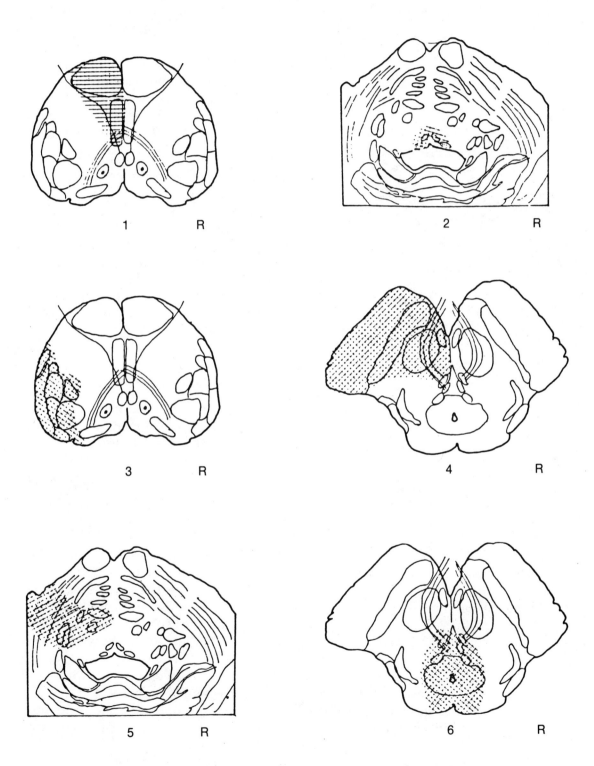

11. Label the cranial nerves and show the destination and function of each.

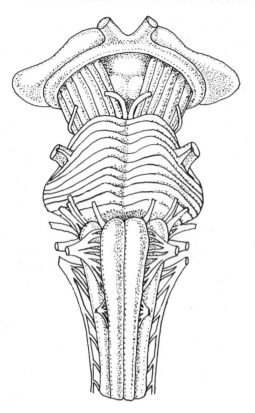

12. Why is a fixed, dilated pupil in an unconscious person an important sign?

CASE HISTORIES

1. Yesterday morning, a 50-year-old man had a sudden onset of diplopia and extreme weakness in the right side of his face, arm, and leg. He stayed in bed for the day and today can walk with his wife's help. His mental status is intact. There is nerve III paralysis on the left side; he is unable to turn the left eye inward, upward, or downward. There is ptosis, or inability to raise the eyelid, of the left lid. The right side of his face droops; he can wrinkle his forehead but when asked to smile, the right side of his lips does not pull back.

Both right arm and leg show a spastic weakness with increased deep tendon reflexes and Babinski's response. There are no sensory deficits.

2. A 56-year-old woman woke up this morning and noticed a pronounced drooping of the left lips and face. Examination showed a decrease in left facial muscle strength on smiling and eye closing. Pain sensation to the face was intact, and the left corneal reflex was sluggish. She could not wrinkle her forehead. Other examination was negative.

3. In a routine employment physical examination on a 36-year-old man, he relates that he has been deaf in his right ear for 3 or 4 years. You confirm this; he cannot "feel" the vibrating tuning fork held to the right mastoid process. When asked to show his teeth, the right corner of his mouth does not draw back fully. He cannot close his right eye tightly, and he has no corneal reflex. All other cranial nerves are intact. Spinal reflexes and muscle strength are intact also.

4. Mr. A. J. reports that his left arm and leg have been clumsy for the last few months. He has trouble picking things up with his left arm. On examination you find a spastic paralysis of the left arm and leg, with hyperreflexia. The left shoulder shows a flaccid weakness with atrophy.

5. H. W. is a 17-year-old high school student who has been bothered by nausea for the last 4 weeks and has lost 10 pounds in this period. He gives as a reason, "I just didn't feel like eating and was overweight anyway." For the last 3 or 4 days the nausea has been much worse and was frequently accompanied by vomiting. On examination, he is oriented to time, place, and person. The only

positive cranial nerve finding is an inability of the left eye to look outward; there is minimal nystagmus in the right eye on inward gaze. Motor strength is good, and reflexes are normal. Finger-to-nose testing shows tremor as does heel-to-shin testing. He walks on a slightly broad base and sways from side to side when standing with his feet close together and eyes closed.

6. A 64-year-old man has had trouble walking for the last five days. He states that about five days ago, "I had a faint spell when working in my garden. I sat down for a few minutes and it passed, but then I noticed my foot dragging." On examination he shows decreased to absent pain response on the entire left side of his body and on both sides of the face. The corneal reflex is absent. There is decreased vibratory sense on the left side of the body. Right-side finger-to-nose testing and heel-to-shin testing show marked side-to-side oscillation. On protrusion, the tongue deviates to the right and there is some atrophy.

7. P. S. is a healthy 8-year-old girl whom you have seen since her birth. Two months ago you saw her because she was occasionally having trouble reading and seeing the print. She also described several episodes of double vision. You were unable to elicit any neurologic abnormalities at that time. Now she has been regurgitating liquids through her nose for the last 4 days, more severely each day. Her mother thinks there has been a change in the quality of her voice in the last week or so. On examination, you find loss of conjugate vision to the right, a uvula that rises slowly and to the left, and atrophy and fasciculation of the tongue, mostly on the right side. There is a minor hearing loss in the right ear. Deep tendon reflexes are brisk on the left side, normal on the right. There is a decrease in pain and temperature sensation and vibratory and position sense on the right side of the body as compared with the left. She has an irregular breathing pattern, combining fairly long periods of not breathing with periods of rapid breathing.

5

Cerebrum

BLOOD SUPPLY TO THE BRAIN

The cells of the brain are completely dependent on a continuous supply of glucose and oxygen. They have meager stores of glycogen and do not carry out glycolysis. If the oxygen supply is cut off, unconsciousness occurs within 30 seconds, and irreversible damage occurs within 5 minutes. Probably the most frequent cause of brain damage is the stoppage of blood flow to a region of the brain, or a *stroke*. Deprived of blood, the cells and axons in the area die and no longer function. If these cells are in the precentral gyrus, voluntary movement of a part of the opposite side of the body is impaired.

All arteries to the brain arise from the aortic arch (Fig. 5-1). The *common carotid arteries* run in the anterior-lateral portion of the neck and can usually be palpated just inside the sternomastoid muscle. Just behind the posterior angle of the jaw, the artery bifurcates into the external and internal carotids. The external carotid supplies the scalp, the dura, and the bones of the skull. The *internal carotid* serves the brain. The carotid bifurcation is a very common site for the

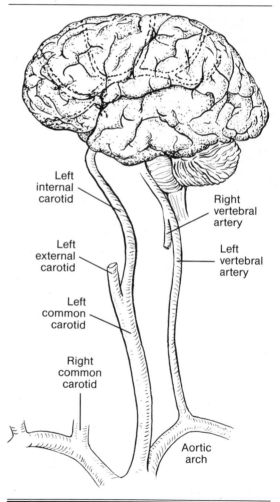

Left internal carotid

Right vertebral artery

Left external carotid

Left vertebral artery

Left common carotid

Right common carotid

Aortic arch

accumulation of *atherosclerotic plaque,* which narrows the artery and reduces blood flow. The narrowing produces a "sush" sound, called a *bruit,* each time the heart beats. Listening with a stethoscope placed over this area often picks up this first and very important sign of arterial narrowing. If neurologic symptoms appear, these narrowings can be removed surgically, usually with excellent return of blood flow.

The two *vertebral arteries* are likewise branches of the aorta. The vertebrals leave the base of the neck and ascend posteriorly to enter the skull through the foramen magnum. Branches supply the medulla and the cerebellum (Fig. 5-2). More superiorly, they join to form the single *basilar artery,* which supplies the pons, midbrain, and parts of the cerebellum. At its superior end the basilar artery branches to form the *posterior cerebral arteries,* which supply the occipital lobes and part of the temporal lobes (Fig. 5-3). In about 20% of us, one (or both) posterior cerebral artery receives most of its blood through the carotid (Figs. 5-4 and 5-5). This whole system forms the *posterior circulation* of the brain.

The *anterior circulation* is supplied by the internal carotid arteries. These arteries enter the cranial cavity and almost immediately branch into middle and anterior cerebral arteries. The *middle cerebral arteries* run through the lateral fissure to supply the lateral surface of the hemispheres. The *anterior cerebral arteries* run anteriorly and medially to loop over the corpus callosum between the hemispheres and to supply blood to the medial surface of the brain (Fig. 5-3).

The anterior and posterior circulations are connected by the *posterior communicating arteries* (Fig. 5-2). The right and left anterior cerebral arteries are connected by the *anterior communicating artery.* Since the carotid and vertebral arteries are interconnected at the base of the brain, a failure of one of these major arteries does not often critically decrease blood flow in the region supplied by

FIGURE 5-2

The cerebral arteries at the base of the brain (seen upside down), their major branches, and the circle of Willis. (From *An Introduction to the Neurosciences.*)

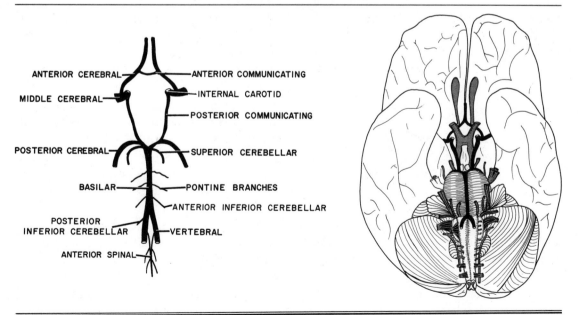

ANTERIOR CEREBRAL
ANTERIOR COMMUNICATING
MIDDLE CEREBRAL
INTERNAL CAROTID
POSTERIOR COMMUNICATING
POSTERIOR CEREBRAL
SUPERIOR CEREBELLAR
BASILAR
PONTINE BRANCHES
ANTERIOR INFERIOR CEREBELLAR
POSTERIOR INFERIOR CEREBELLAR
VERTEBRAL
ANTERIOR SPINAL

F I G U R E 5-3
The territories perfused by the anterior, middle, and posterior cerebral arteries on the lateral surface of the cerebrum.

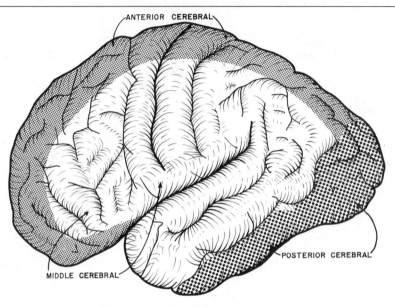

that vessel. The interconnection of these arteries forms a circle first described by the eminent English anatomist, Thomas Willis. It is consequently called the *circle of Willis* in his honor.

These arteries can be studied by injecting an x-ray–opaque dye from a catheter inserted in the femoral artery and guided up the aorta to the origin of the desired vessel. Figure 5-4 shows an angiogram taken in the lateral view, while Figure 5-5 was taken in the anterior-posterior view.

Cerebrovascular Disease

Transient Ischemic Attacks (TIAs). Focal loss of neurologic function for a few minutes, usually caused by low blood flow (ischemia) to that region, is called a transient ischemic attack (TIA). TIAs usually have an abrupt onset and slower resolution. The first few TIAs rarely leave neurologic deficits, but multiple TIAs often do. They are usually caused by a severe stenosis of a major artery, such as stenosis of the bifurcation of the carotid. (The case of Mr. J. H. on page 102 is an example.) Treatment with antiplatelet drugs such as aspirin seems to reduce the likelihood of TIAs progressing into strokes.

Cessation of the blood supply to all or part of the central nervous system (CNS) is called a stroke or cerebral vascular accident (CVA). It is the most common affliction of the nervous system and a leading cause of death. Strokes also cause much disability; perhaps as many as a third of all disabled older patients have had strokes. The two major types of CVAs are infarction and intracerebral hemorrhage.

Infarction. Plugging any blood vessel of the brain deprives that region of glucose and oxygen. The mechanism of plugging is variable. Fatty, white plaque may develop inside the arteries to reduce blood flow. Some of this plaque breaks free to plug vessels elsewhere. Other plaque serves as sites for platelet aggregation or blood clot formation. This causes plugging either at that site or further up after the aggregate or clot breaks free. In any case, brain tissue is deprived of blood flow and an ischemic infarct occurs. Other than the acute loss of neurologic function, there are few reliable signs of the onset of infarction; less than half of all patients lose consciousness. The ischemic area usually shows on computerized tomography (CT) and magnetic resonance imaging (MRI) scans.

After the initial ischemia, the region becomes edematous, or swells, as cells die and leak their contents. Often a much larger region is transiently nonfunctional because of this swelling. The infarcted region becomes necrotic 3 to 7 days later. White blood cells and microglia move in to phagocytize the dead cells. The swelling gradually subsides. Three months later the region has shrunk and is filled with connective tissue.

Atherothrombic infarcts in the brain are uncommon before age 50 but increase in frequency thereafter. Previous transient ischemic attacks, other clinical evidence of atherosclerosis, and high blood lipids are predisposing factors for these infarcts. High blood pressure is a secondary risk factor. Death within 1 week occurs in less than a quarter of patients with a major brain vessel occluded. The symptoms are most severe immediately after the stroke, but the rate of recovery is hard to predict. The earlier motor function, even spasticity, returns, the more hopeful the prognosis.

About half of the stroke patients who survive are permanently disabled. Reduction of risk factors such as hypertension, hyperlipidemia, smoking, and diabetes have reduced the incidence of stroke in the last 10 years. Long-term aspirin therapy remains controversial. Acute therapy for clot lysis, which now shows such promising results in coronary thrombosis, is a much more difficult therapy in the cerebral circulation. This is because ischemic and hemorrhagic infarcts are frequently very difficult to tell apart. Prudence suggests doing a computerized tomography (CT) scan to rule out hemorrhage before starting clot lysis therapy; yet it is early therapy that has proved so valuable in treating myocardial infarcts.

Atherosclerosis may also cause widespread arterial narrowing and multiple small strokes—known as *lacunar strokes*—which can result in greatly impaired mental capacity ("feeblemindedness") instead of a catastrophic episode.

Embolic infarcts occur at an earlier age, and indeed are not rare in childhood. The left side of the heart is a major source of the emboli, which are often blood clots.

General personality changes are common in patients who have suffered strokes. They often change mood rapidly, crying one minute, laughing the next, and sometimes remaining depressed for days. Patients with a left-sided (dominant) stroke often have language disturbances, and communication with them is sometimes possible only through gestures. Many such patients go through a phase of saying only "No!" Relearning is hampered by the communication difficulty as well as by a slow, cautious behavior style. These patients need a great deal of feedback, often at each step. They may have a problem with memory. Patients with a nondominant lesion often show neglect for their left side and have much difficulty with spacial-perceptual tasks. They are usually unaware of these difficulties since they tend to have a quick and impulsive personality style after the stroke.

F I G U R E 5-4
Right carotid arteriogram *(opposite)* seen in a lateral view, that is, looking over the patient's right shoulder at the right side of the head. A x-ray–opaque dye was injected into the carotid. The internal carotid artery is identified by the *large arrow.* Just after entering the cranial cavity, the internal carotid branches into the posterior communicating artery *(two arrows),* which feeds the posterior cerebral artery *(three arrows).* This pattern of the posterior cerebral artery receiving blood from the internal carotid is fairly common. After making a further twist, the internal carotid branches into the anterior cerebral artery *(four arrows)* and into the middle cerebral artery, which traverses the lateral fissure. This portion of the artery is pointing straight at the observer and is hard to see. The surface branches of the middle cerebral artery are marked by single arrows. (Arteriogram courtesy of Robert Wright, M.D., St. Francis Medical Center, Peoria, IL.)

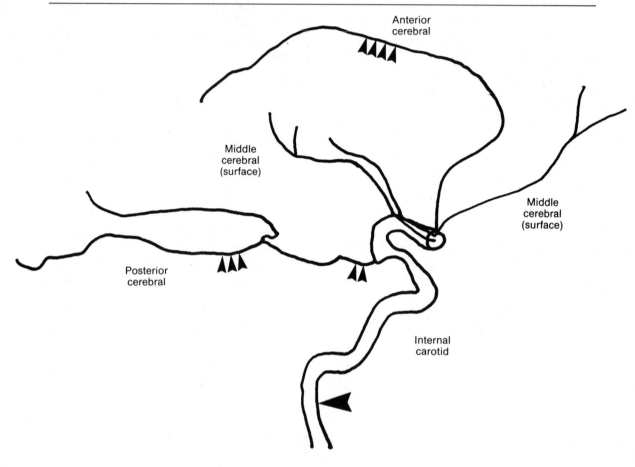

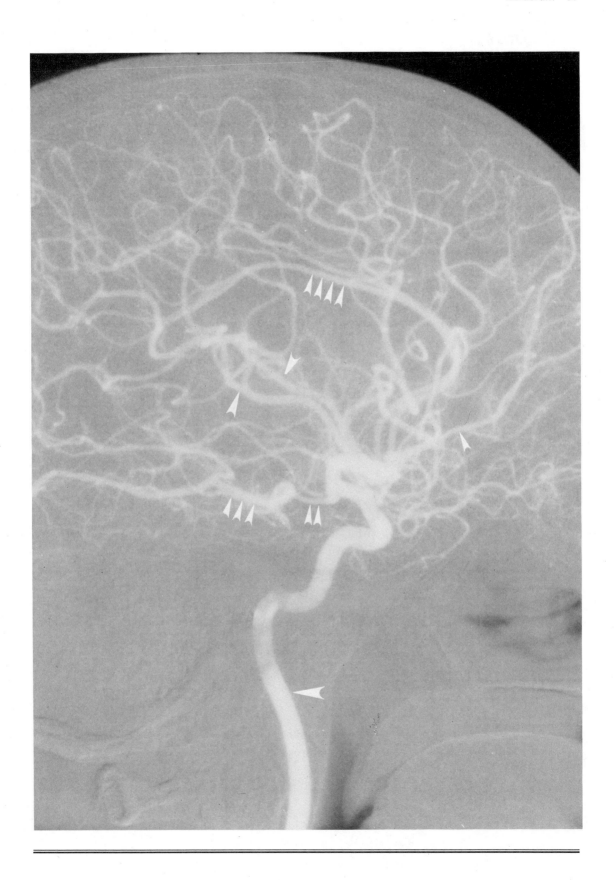

F I G U R E 5-5

The same arteriogram as Figure 5-4, seen in an anterior-posterior (AP) view (as if you were looking through the patient's forehead). The internal carotid artery *(large arrow)* branches into the posterior communicating artery *(two arrows),* the middle cerebral artery *(single small arrow),* and the anterior cerebral artery *(four arrows).* The contralateral anterior cerebral artery is filling with dye through the anterior communicating artery. The posterior communicating artery *(two arrows)* feeds the posterior cerebral artery *(three arrows).* (Arteriogram courtesy of Robert Wright, M.D., St. Francis Medical Center, Peoria, IL.)

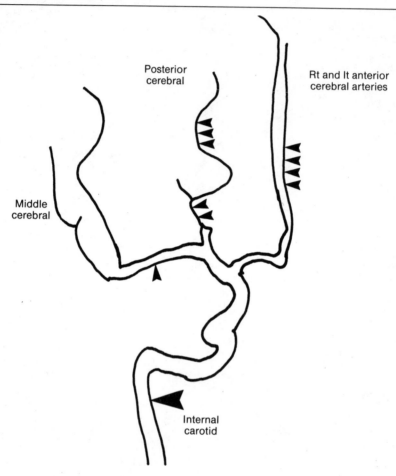

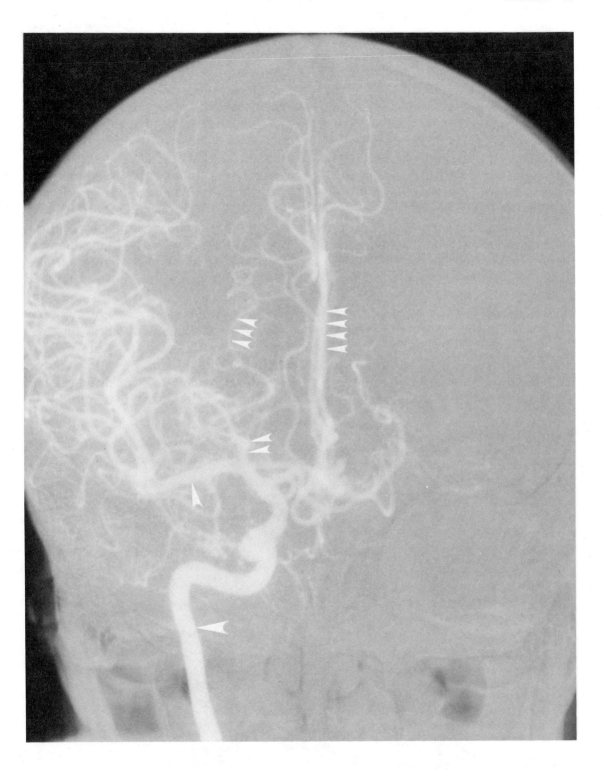

Hemorrhage. Leakage of blood within the skull causes many neurologic problems, largely because the skull has a fixed size. The addition of an intercranial mass of blood compresses the brain. The compressed brain area ceases to function and brings on direct neurologic findings such as hemiplegia. Further expansion of the pool of blood causes the brain to seek more room and to herniate through the tentorium.

Intracerebral hemorrhage results from the rupture of a cerebral vessel, often in the internal capsule region (Fig. 5-6). In addition to an ischemic area, there is a large-space–occupying blood clot. This often causes a headache before increasing intracranial pressure leads to nausea, vomiting, and often unconsciousness. Many patients die within 1 to 3 days after an intracerebral hemorrhage. Surgical removal of the clot is often pos-sible. Hypertension is a major risk factor. Hemorrhagic infarcts are uncommon before the age of 40.

Extradural hematomas are caused by bleeding from any of the arteries feeding the dural covering of the brain. These hematomas cause a large blood mass to press on the brain. Such pressure causes cessation of brain function under the clot. Extradural hematomas are almost always the result of trauma; history and examination of the skull usually confirm this diagnosis. Typically, the patient is unconscious for a few minutes at the time of injury, regains consciousness, is clear and lucid for a few hours, and then rapidly becomes sleepy, or unconscious, with a developing hemiplegia and dilated pupils. Unless these signs are correctly interpreted and the clot removed, extradural hematomas are usually fatal. For this reason every patient with a

F I G U R E 5-6
CT scan of the head showing an intracerebral hemorrhage. (Courtesy of George Zwicky, M.D., St. Francis Medical Center, Peoria, IL.)

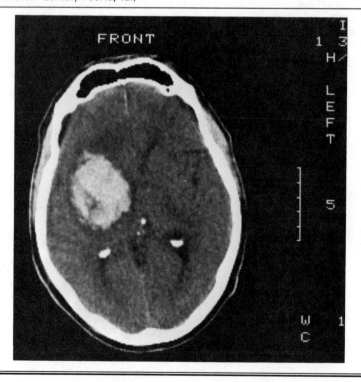

head injury should be suspected of having an extradural hematoma, and any lapse into sleepiness or unconsciousness should be cause for concern. A CT scan is a rapid and accurate diagnostic test.

Subdural hematomas are caused by venous bleeding into the space between the dura and the brain. The relation of subdural hematomas to trauma is much less clear; days or weeks usually elapse between injury or symptoms.

FRONTAL LOBES

Primary Motor Cortex

The final cortical pathway for voluntary motor control begins on the precentral gyrus (see Fig. 1-6). From this area come the commands for all our fine motor movements, such as opposing the thumb to the palm of the hand or flexing an individual finger to the palm. Discrete stimulation here gives only individual muscle movement.

The area of motor cortex devoted to each region of the body is not uniform (Fig. 5-7). The motor cortex controlling the face and hand occupies nearly two-thirds of the precentral gyrus. This distribution seems to be related to the complexity of movement the body area carries out. Semiautomatic movements such as walking require very little of the motor area to start the pattern, while the fine, delicate movements of the face and hands occupy a great deal of area.

Another way of describing the allotment of motor areas is to consider types of movements largely limited to primates, such as finger and toe flexion and facial expression. These motor commands originate in the precentral gyrus, travel in the corticospinal and corticobulbar tracts, and reach the contralateral motor nuclei of the brain stem and the contralateral anterior horn cells of the

F I G U R E 5-7
The motor representation of the body on the precentral gyrus. This homunculus is arranged over the surface of a coronal section of a cerebral hemisphere. Note the large area devoted to the hand and face.

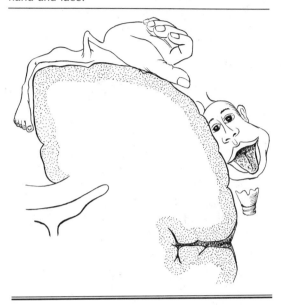

spinal cord with rarely more than one interneuron in between. Destruction of the precentral gyrus alone seriously impairs, if it does not destroy, the fine movements of the hand and face while leaving grosser movement patterns, such as walking, much less impaired.

The organization of body areas on the motor cortex can be seen by studying the spreading electrical activity of a motor seizure. The patient may begin a fit with a twitching in the left leg; this twitching spreads from the leg to the trunk, into the hand, and finally into the face. These are called *Jacksonian seizures.*

Rapid destruction of the motor cortex, as by a stroke, results first in a flaccid paralysis. This changes in 2 to 6 weeks to the classic spastic paralysis of the upper motor neuron syndrome: weakness, hyperreflexia, increased tone, and Babinski's sign. The sooner spasticity returns the more likely that function, if not fine movement, will return.

Transient Ischemic Attacks of Hand Area

Mr. J. H. is a 62-year-old obese white male who complains of spells "when his hand goes to sleep." These episodes last for 5 to 10 minutes, began occurring about 4 years ago, and have occurred after almost every meal for the last couple of weeks. During these spells his right wrist drops, and he has trouble moving his right hand and forearm. If he pinches his right hand during this time, he cannot feel it. Examination reveals reduction of the pulse of the left carotid, of the right radial, and of the right dorsalis pedis. There is a loud bruit in the left neck. There is reduction in pinprick and position sense in the right hand, with a slightly more active right biceps reflex. Otherwise, review of systems and physical examination are normal.

A left carotid arteriogram shows a marked narrowing of both the common carotid and the internal carotid, particularly at the bifurcation. A left carotid endarterectomy, or reaming out of the carotid, is done. A low-fat diet is given to help him lose weight and to reduce the formation of atherosclerotic plaque. Two years after the procedure, he has had no further attacks and has lost 50 pounds.

This case history provides a good example of a brain region not receiving its needed supply of blood and not functioning as a result. Whenever arterial pressure falls, the capillaries at the ends of its arterial tree suffer most. In this case the distant capillaries of the middle and anterior cerebral arteries are most affected. The hand area of the precentral gyrus is particularly vulnerable since it receives blood from the ends of both the middle and anterior cerebral arteries (see Fig. 5-3). Transient ischemic attacks are frequently followed by total occlusion of the blood supply, with grave consequences.

Premotor Area

The premotor or *supplemental motor area* (See Fig. 1-6) teams up with the precentral gyrus to produce integrated motor movement. An example of this type of coordination is found in the premotor eye field high in the hemisphere. Stimulation here results in a coordinated turning of both the head and eyes. The function of the premotor area is to initiate coordinated movements rather than to initiate individual muscle movements as does the motor cortex.

Lesions in the premotor area give an unsteady quality to walking without the classic upper motor neuron signs. Lesions here also allow a more complex reflex, namely a *grasp*, to be elicited. As you know, when a baby's palm is stroked with a pencil, it reflexively flexes its fingers to grasp the object. As the baby develops, this reflex disappears because it is inhibited from the premotor cortex. Return of the grasp reflex in an adult suggests loss of this inhibition due to dysfunction of the anterior-frontal lobe.

Prefrontal Area

The prefrontal area operates in conjunction with many deeper areas of the cerebrum and diencephalon to modulate our outlook on life and our behavior patterns. Patients with frontal lobe damage are usually apathetic and care little about their appearance or surroundings. A previously meticulous housekeeper becomes a slovenly, unwashed person who rarely bothers to eat and is never interested in keeping up her house. Other generalized nervous diseases attack the prefrontal areas and lead to dementia. Alzheimer's disease is an example.

Personality Change

R. J., a 17-year-old high-school student, had a straight-A average, played basketball, and was student council president. Six months ago he began acting strangely and impulsively and rapidly became an outcast. Street drugs were implicated, but urine screening was negative. Antipsychotic drug therapy calmed him down, but he could not function in school and lived at a psychiatric facility. One month ago he became violent and had to be restrained or kept in a padded room for 2 to 3 weeks. When he had calmed down enough to keep his head in the machine, he was studied by an MRI scan. A large, highly vascular, encapsulated subfrontal mass was resected, and his behavior returned to normal in 2 months. The possibility of recurrence of this *meningioma* is very low, and meningiomas rarely metastasize.

PARIETAL LOBES

Primary Sensory Cortex

The representation of the body surface on the postcentral gyrus is similar to that of the motor cortex (Fig. 5-7). All the primary modalities (pain and temperature, vibration and position sense, and touch) are represented here.

After rapid destruction of the postcentral gyrus, *hemianesthesia* develops; there is no sensation on the opposite side of the body. In a few days to weeks, pain sensation returns to near normal. A patient's ability to tell where the pain is applied is usually limited to the hand or forearm but not to smaller areas. It is thought that the thalamus takes over the job as the primary sensory area for pain when the parietal lobe is destroyed. Other primary sensory modalities recover more slowly to about half their previous sensitivity.

Sensory Association Areas

The more posterior portion of each parietal lobe uses primary sensory inputs from the postcentral gyrus to reach higher-order sensory discrimination.

These sensory association areas allow us to discriminate between pinpricks caused by one pin or by two pins held close together. This ability is called *two-point discrimination*. Naming coins placed in the hand (*stereogenesis*) or numbers drawn on the palm (*graphesthesia*) are other examples.

The function of the remainder of the right and left parietal lobes is vastly different. The dominant (usually left) parietal lobe is the central point for language integration and will be discussed in Chapter 7. The nondominant lobe is a vast area with few known functions. Among them is awareness of the opposite side of the body. Lesions in the nondominant lobe result in a patient who forgets to button the left cuff or even to put on the left shoe. These patients often have a curious denial of illness. Even though they have impaired vision and movement, patients with a tumor centered in the nondominant lobe steadfastly deny that anything is wrong and often refuse surgery.

TEMPORAL LOBES

Discussion of the function of the temporal lobes is complicated by the presence, deep within each lobe, of part of a much older and very primitive visceral brain whose functions are very poorly understood. Most disease processes affecting the temporal lobe cortex usually spread to this deeper structure, part of the limbic system (see Fig. 7-2).

The *primary auditory cortex* lies inside the lateral fissure. To see it, a temporal lobe must be pulled down (see Fig. 1-3). Neurons from both ears end here. Realization of sounds in either ear occurs here. In the dominant hemisphere, the area surrounding the primary cortex is involved in interpreting sounds as words. Vestibular sensations are also projected onto the temporal lobes.

The remainder of the temporal lobes seems to involve memory storage. Temporal lobe seizures often result in hallucinations involving previous experiences. Such seizures may involve any of the senses. Olfactory hallucinations commonly occur as part of a temporal lobe seizure. The odor imagined is usually described as a very unpleasant, but unfamiliar, one.

OCCIPITAL LOBES

The *primary visual cortex*, located on the medial surface of each occipital lobe, receives the projection of the contralateral visual fields (see Fig. 4-19). The cells of this lobe "see" the world as a collection of short lines that have different spatial orientations, lengths, and colors. To stimulate the visual cortex effectively, an observed object must be moving or flashing. A truly stationary image quickly disappears from a person's view. Building these colored lines into language is the function of the rest of the dominant occipital lobe. Seizures of the occipital lobe give illusions of brightly colored simple patterns, such as red wavy lines on a blue background.

DEEPER CEREBRAL STRUCTURES

Horizontal Sections

Sectioning a brain in a plane parallel with the ears and the nose (Fig. 5-8) results in a horizontal section (Figs. 5-9, 5-10, and 5-11). Several structures seen in these sections have already been discussed. The *thalamus* (Fig. 5-9) is buried deep within the cerebrum. The *corpus callosum* is seen only in the anterior part of the section because its midportion has an upward curve (Fig. 5-8).

Notice that the cerebrum is divided into white matter (myelinated axons) on the inside and gray matter (cell bodies) on the outside. The extensive convolutions of the brain's outer gray matter provide an enormous surface area for the integrative action of the brain.

There are two large collections of cell bodies (nuclei) lying between the thalamus and the gray matter of the cortex. They are jointly referred to as *basal nuclei*. The *caudate nucleus* is the more anterior and medial, while the *lenticular nucleus* is more lateral. Both these nuclei are part of the motor system and serve to modify and amplify rather than to initiate movement.

The tract (white matter) separating the thalamus and caudate nucleus from the lenticular nucleus is the *internal capsule*. All fibers leaving the precentral gyrus and the other motor areas of the frontal lobe flow through the internal capsule on their way to the brain stem and spinal cord. The corticospinal and corticobulbar tracts flow through the internal capsule.

A second MRI scan in a horizontal section is shown in Figure 5-12. This section is above the corpus callosum and shows the white and gray matter of the two cerebral hemispheres. The cleft between the two hemispheres is the *interhemispheric fissure*. The anterior cerebral arteries lie in this fissure.

C A S E   H I S T O R Y
Stroke to Internal Capsule–Thalamus Area

Ms. J. M., a 48-year-old banker who had atrial flutter, was presiding at a board of directors meeting when she stopped talking in midsentence, slumped in her chair, had a mild left-sided seizure, and lost consciousness. She remained unconscious for 48 hours with flaccid paralysis and areflexia on the entire left side. Her pupils reacted briskly to light. One week later she still could not move her left face, arm, or leg, which all became hyperreflexic. She

The solid line shows the plane of the horizontal section in Figures 5-9, 5-10, and 5-11. The dotted line shows the plane of the coronal section shown in Figures 5-13, 5-14, and 5-15. (From *An Introduction to the Neurosciences.*)

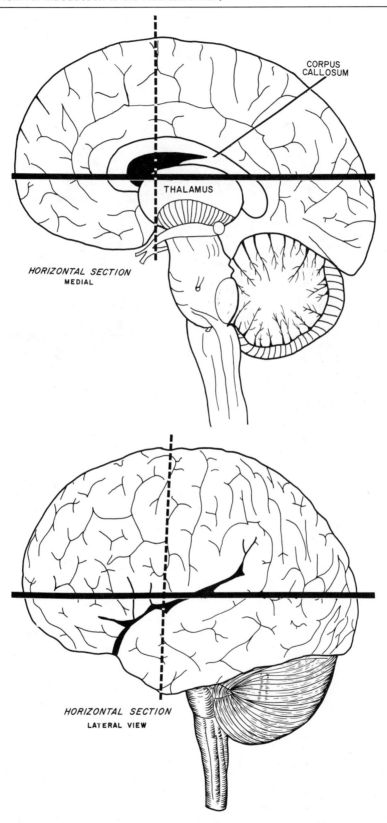

CORPUS CALLOSUM

THALAMUS

HORIZONTAL SECTION
MEDIAL

HORIZONTAL SECTION
LATERAL VIEW

F I G U R E 5-9
Horizontal section of a human brain through the thalamus, internal capsule, and basal
ganglia region.

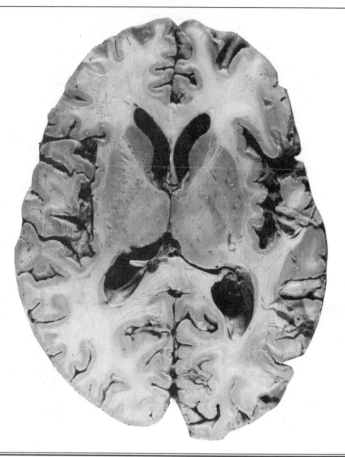

was unable to feel pinprick or other sensation on the left side and was unable to see in the left visual field. Her speech was clear and coherent.

Expressing a great desire to "get up and around," she started occupational and physical therapy in the second week. Strength in the left shoulder and hip rapidly improved. She was walking on bars at the end of the third week, with a walker at the end of the fourth week, and unassisted during the sixth week. Her walk was halting; she swung her left leg out (circumducting gait) rather than lifting it. The visual deficit cleared. She could appreciate sensation in her left side but not locate it precisely. She could not identify coins or numbers drawn on her left hand.

Over the next 2 months the facial paralysis gradually cleared and she could walk more easily, if not more gracefully. Her left shoulder was strong. Her left hand, arm, and forearm had hyperactive reflexes but no voluntary motion. Her gait continued to be circumducting. She returned to work, part-time, 4 months after the stroke and resumed full-time work after 6 months.

The initial event, clearly of sudden onset, was probably caused by embolic material from the left auricle that plugged a cerebral artery. This is an ischemic (bloodless) stroke. Because

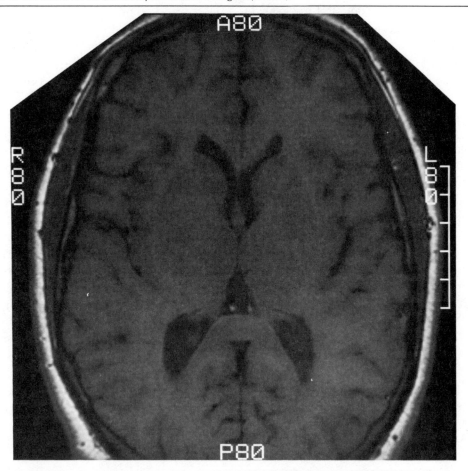

F I G U R E 5-11
Labeled drawing of Figure 5-9.

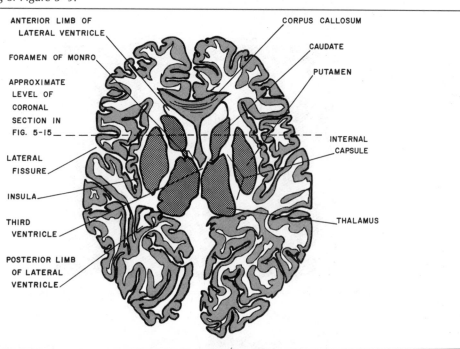

ANTERIOR LIMB OF
LATERAL VENTRICLE

FORAMEN OF MONRO

APPROXIMATE
LEVEL OF
CORONAL
SECTION IN
FIG. 5-15

LATERAL
FISSURE

INSULA

THIRD
VENTRICLE

POSTERIOR LIMB
OF LATERAL
VENTRICLE

CORPUS CALLOSUM

CAUDATE

PUTAMEN

INTERNAL
CAPSULE

THALAMUS

of the loss of voluntary control of the left side of her face, arm, and leg; because of her sensory loss in the same areas; and because of her visual loss, the ischemic area was located in the right internal capsule-thalamus area. As the pupils reacted briskly to light, an intercerebral hemorrhage was unlikely.

Interruption of the anterior cerebral artery would have paralyzed her leg and hand, while interruption of the middle cerebral artery would have paralyzed her hand and face. Only in the internal capsule area does plugging of a single artery give paralysis of the face, arm, and leg. The thalamus lying just medial to the internal capsule is initially involved in J. M.'s problem. The visual pathway, on its path from the posterior-inferior thalamus to the occipital lobe, arches close to the internal capsule.

Coronal Sections

When the brain is sectioned vertically, as if through both ears, a coronal section is formed. The lines of cut are shown by the dashed lines in Figure 5-8. The resulting section is shown in Figures 5-13 through 5-15. The cerebral cortex is a cellular layer on the outer surface of the cerebrum. Under the layer is a huge mass of white matter (myelinated axons), which connects the cortex to the body and, just as important, one cortical region to another. It is probably fair to say that every cerebral area connects to every other cerebral area and, by the *corpus callosum*, to the other side of the cerebrum as well. The internal capsule carries all information leaving the cerebrum on its way to lower structures. The corticospinal tract is one of the more important of the many fiber tracts here.

Lying around the internal capsule are the *basal nuclei*. These structures act in concert with the motor cortex to produce harmonious, graceful movements and are involved in coordinating such

F I G U R E 5-12
Axial MRI scan at a more superior level than Figure 5-10. This MRI shows the characteristic multiple high signal (bright) patches of multiple sclerosis. (Courtesy of Gerald Palagallo, M.D.)

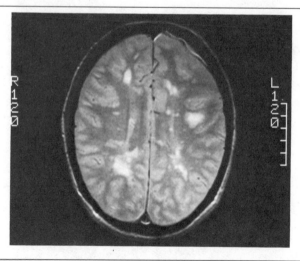

complex acts as walking. The *thalamus* is seen lying on either side of the third ventricle. These two structures are fed by short vertical branches of the middle cerebral artery and are especially prone to hemorrhage after long-standing hypertension.

Two more MRI scans in the coronal plane are shown in Figures 5-16 and 5-17.

Ventricular System

Now that you can recognize the major structures of the brain in both horizontal and coronal planes, you are ready to picture a structure in three dimensions. The ventricular system is composed of cavelike structures deep within the brain that are filled with cerebrospinal fluid. Ventricles developed during evolution as the brain folded on itself several times to accommodate the increasing size of the cerebrum. These foldings now occur during embryological development.

The *lateral ventricles* (Fig. 5-18) lie in the cerebrum and are the largest of the ventricles. The horizontal section (shown in Fig. 5-9) cuts through the lateral ventricles as shown in Figure 5-19. The connection between the anterior and posterior horns lies above the plane of the section. Remember that the lateral ventricles, like the cerebral hemispheres in which they lie, are bilateral. Both lateral ventricles connect with a single midline structure, the third ventricle. The *third ventricle* lies between the two halves of the diencephalon and is connected to a midline structure, the *fourth ventricle,* by means of the *cerebral aqueduct.* The fourth ventricle lies between the brain stem and the cerebellum.

Cerebrospinal fluid is produced in the lateral ventricles and flows through the third and fourth ventricles. It leaves the fourth ventricle, flows around the outside of the brain, and is reabsorbed by a large venous sinus at the top of the brain. The brain floats in the cerebrospinal fluid surrounding it.

Blockage of the flow of cerebrospinal fluid leads to *hydrocephalus.* A common point of blockage in children is the cerebral aqueduct between the third and fourth ventricles. The lateral ventricles enlarge and press the brain tissue against the skull. If the sutures of the skull have not closed, as is usually the case in children less than 2 years old, the skull expands rapidly. This condition can be treated by running a draining shunt from a lateral ventricle into the abdominal cavity.

Enlargement of the lateral ventricles occurs with age and probably reflects the continuous loss of neurons with age. Many patients with dementia have enlarged ventricles, indicating extensive loss of neurons. Some of these patients benefit from shunting cerebrospinal fluid out of the ventricles.

Except in children less than 2 years old, the skull is a rigid structure. Any expanding mass within the skull, such as a tumor or a hemorrhage, increases *intercranial pressure.* We have already discussed the role of increased intercranial pressure in producing its cardinal sign, papilledema. Other early signs include nausea and vomiting as a result of pressure on the medulla. Diplopia is often a result of pressure on the sixth cranial nerve. Intercranial pressure can be measured by a spinal tap but should be done with great caution if papilledema is present. If the flow of fluid is partially blocked, removing fluid from the lower spinal cord can cause herniation of the medial temporal lobe or the cerebellum.

F I G U R E 5-13
Coronal section of the brain at the level of the optic chiasm.

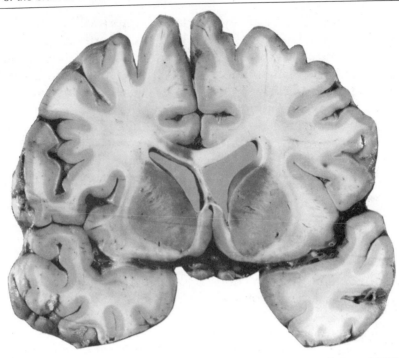

F I G U R E 5-14
MRI scan at the same level. (Courtesy of Gerald Palagallo, M.D.)

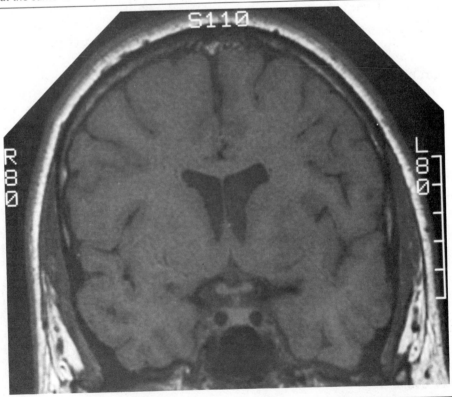

FIGURE 5-15
Labeled drawing of Figure 5-13.

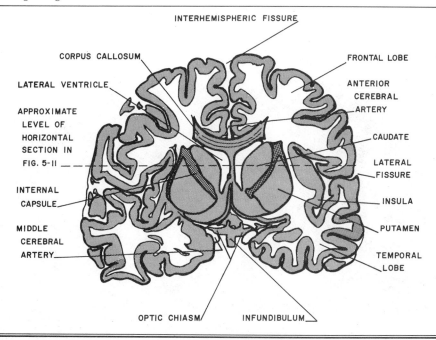

FIGURE 5-16
Coronal MRI scan through the thalamus. The plane of section is shown in Figure 9-2. (Courtesy of Gerald Palagallo, M.D.)

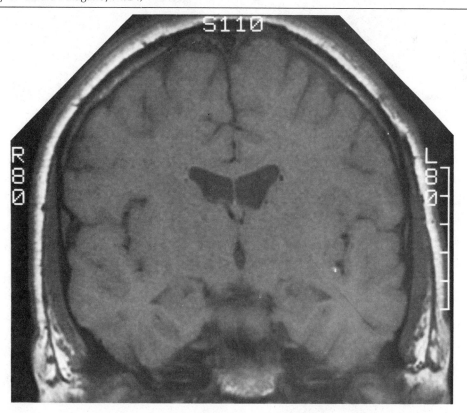

F I G U R E 5-17
Coronal MRI scan at the junction of the occipital lobes with the parietal and temporal lobes. (Courtesy of Gerald Palagallo, M.D.)

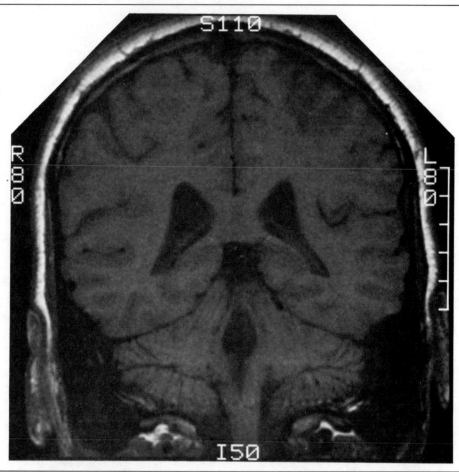

OTHER DISEASES

Headache

Over 80% of the population will suffer one or more headaches this year. The brain itself contains no pain or other sensory endings, but the larger blood vessels running into the brain do contain pain endings, as does the dura. Probably two-thirds of all headaches are *muscle tension headaches*, characterized by a bilateral gripping sensation around the forehead and the base of the skull. Prolonged contraction of these muscles is the usual cause. Tension headaches are relieved by time, aspirin, or acetaminophen.

Migraine headaches are more severe, occur in 10 to 20% of the population, and are three times more common in females. They usually start in childhood. The throbbing pain, usually on one side

F I G U R E 5-18
Ventricular system of the brain shown in lateral **(A)** and **(B)** anterior-posterior view.
(From *An Introduction to the Neurosciences.*)

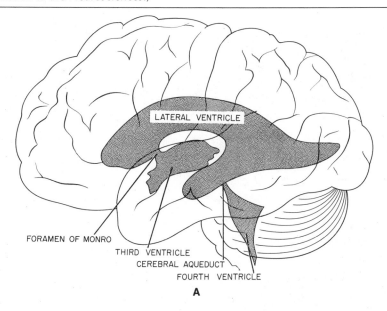

LATERAL VENTRICLE

FORAMEN OF MONRO

THIRD VENTRICLE
CEREBRAL AQUEDUCT
FOURTH VENTRICLE

A

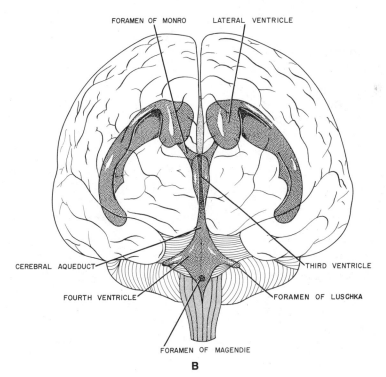

FORAMEN OF MONRO   LATERAL VENTRICLE

CEREBRAL AQUEDUCT

FOURTH VENTRICLE

THIRD VENTRICLE

FORAMEN OF LUSCHKA

FORAMEN OF MAGENDIE

B

F I G U R E 5-19
The plane, through a lateral view of the ventricular system, of the horizontal section in Figure 5-9.

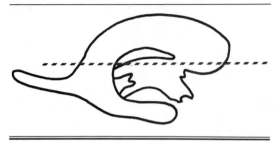

of the head, has a sudden onset. The pain may last for hours or occasionally days. Some sufferers will have a transient symptom, an aura, such as "seeing flashing lights," before the onset of the headache. These headaches are caused by the dilatation of the arteries in the skull and brain. They can often be treated by vasoconstrictive drugs.

Cluster headaches occur primarily in middle-aged men and exhibit a burning, searing, stabbing pain centered or pointed toward the orbit of the eye. They often occur at night. The pain is frequently excruciating and usually lasts an hour or so.

Headache may occasionally be a sign of generalized increased intercranial pressure. These headaches are usually described as dull and diffuse and are not localized in one area of the head. The headache of increased intercranial pressure is usually worse on arising.

Only a very small fraction of all headaches herald serious intracranial disease, yet the possibility should not be overlooked. Such headaches are usually different from and more severe than a patient's previous headache pattern. Patients can usually localize the pain; it is persistent and does not respond to aspirin or vasoconstrictive drugs. The presence of focal neurologic signs should be a tip-off for an extensive workup.

A headache "worse than anything I have ever felt" can frequently be a sign of a small bleed into the subdural space, usually from a leaking aneurysm. These patients often have a stiff neck, which is secondary to irritated brain coverings caused by blood in the subarachnoid space.

C A S E   H I S T O R Y
A Crushing Headache

Ms. D. F. had the sudden onset of a crushing headache, which she describes as "the worst headache I have ever had and different than any other." Her right eye deviated out, and the right pupil was dilated. A CT scan showed blood around the base of the brain. The right carotid angiogram in Figure 5-20 shows an aneurysm of the right posterior communicating artery. The aneurysm was clipped to prevent the occurrence of rebleeding, which is common and frequently fatal.

Stiff Neck

Patients hold the neck rigid because of great pain on movement. The coverings of the brain, including the dura, are inflamed or irritated. If patients have other signs of a bacterial infection such as fever, chills, and malaise, the cause is probably *bacterial meningitis*. This disease can be treated with antibiotics with low morbidity or mortality. *Viral encephalitis* causes malaise and joint pain as well as a stiff neck. Antiviral therapy is helpful as is supportive therapy, including fluids.

Seizures

The brain functions by the orderly passage of minute electrical signals along functionally meaningful path-

F I G U R E 5-20
Angiogram showing an aneurysm of the right posterior communicating artery. (Courtesy of Terry Brady, M.D., St. Francis Medical Center, Peoria, IL.)

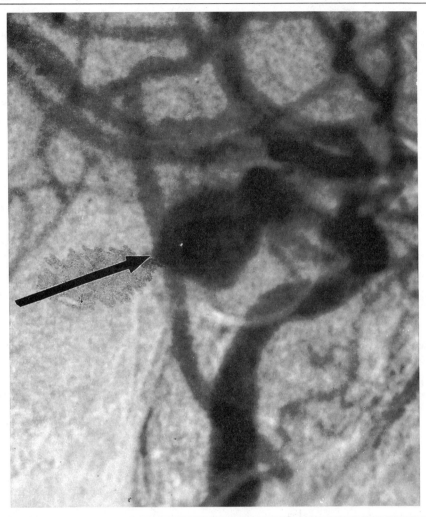

ways. These signals are usually initiated by sensation from the outside world.

At times, and often for obscure causes, electrical signals originating within the brain grow larger and spread in pathways that have little or no functional meaning. As they spread, these electrical signals activate brain neurons and result in seizures. Seizures may involve only a motor component (such as a jerky movement of the hand), only a sensory component (such as a horrible smell), or behavior modification. Sometimes the causative focus is an irritation to the brain, such as a tumor edge or a scar in the dura. Often no "organic" focus can be found, and we hide our ignorance with the term *epilepsy*.

Epilepsy is a chronic disease that afflicts roughly 1% of the population. Excessive abnormal neural activity of a seizure is often expressed in the cerebral cortex. This abnormal activity can be measured by scalp recordings of the electrical activity of brain. Electroencephalography (EEG) plays an important role in the diagnosis and treatment of the various forms of epilepsy.

Simple partial seizures may be expressed behaviorally by a twitching of the hand, which then spreads to twitching of the whole arm. Partial seizures may occur in any lobe and cause problems appropriate to that lobe; for example, focal seizures of the occipital lobe cause patients to see flashing lights and wavy lines. If the seizure is in the frontal or anterior temporal lobe, confused behavior may be the only overt sign. Simple partial seizures can also be caused by gross pathology, such as a tumor, which would also cause neurologic signs. High fever, particularly in children, may cause simple partial seizures.

Complex partial seizures are similar to simple partial seizures but lead to impairment of consciousness.

In *generalized tonic clonic* (grand mal) *seizures,* patients may experience an aura or hallucination a few seconds before they lose consciousness and undergo 1 to 2 minutes of massive muscle movement. These movements are usually cyclic and usually involve all the body muscles. Biting the tongue, cheeks, or both is common, but attempts to prevent it usually make matters worse.

After the motor portion of the seizure, patients remain unconscious for up to an hour and then often sleep for several hours. On awakening, patients are aware that the seizure has occurred. These attacks can begin at any age and may recur either the next day or the next year. The frequency and duration of tonic clonic seizures can increase, decrease, or remain constant over the succeeding years.

Drug therapy for these three types of seizures includes carbamazepine (Tegretol), phenytoin (Dilantin), and valproate (Depakene). They may cause drowsiness and interfere with cognitive function to varying degrees but not to the degree associated with phenobarbital, an old standby in the treatment of seizures.

Absence (petit mal) *seizures* are most common in children and are a 20 to 30 second interruption of attentiveness. The child rarely falls or otherwise shows signs of seizures, which frequently occur many times a day. The child stares blankly at a random area for the period of the seizure. Seizures may occur so often that they affect the child's performance in school. Ethosuximide (Zarontin) and valproate (Depakene) are useful drugs in the treatment of petit mal seizures.

Status epilepticus is a state of continuous seizure activity lasting longer than 5 minutes. Intravenous diazepam is the drug of choice.

Many factors may bring on seizures in susceptible persons. Flashing lights or a rolling television screen are sometimes the cause. Hyperventilation or long periods of sleeplessness are especially likely to bring on seizures.

CASE HISTORY
Seizure in Shoulder-Leg Area

This 37-year-old, right-handed steel mill employee experienced episodes of repetitive jerks of his shoulder (simple partial seizures). The episodes lasted a few seconds and occurred once every few days. These episodes occurred without warning and initially did not involve the face, hand, or legs. No weakness was present.

A month later, the patient had two prolonged episodes of uncontrollable jerking of his left shoulder and arm, which spread down to the fingers of the left hand, and progressed to unconsciousness (complex partial seizures). The patient continued to have simple partial seizures involving the left arm with clenching and jerking of his left hand despite treatment with anticonvulsants (phenobarbital and phenytoin).

After several of these complex partial seizures, a transient weakness and hyperreflexia of his left leg developed. An MRI scan showed a mass on the right side, high in the frontal-parietal lobe junction. At surgery a relatively superficial but intrinsic tumor, 4 to 5 cm in diameter, was found. The tumor contained areas of necrosis and a base of cystic cavities. Cortex, white matter, and tumor were resected until white matter of apparently normal appearance was encountered. Pathologic examination of the tumor indicated a very malignant tumor of glial tissue: a glioblastoma multiforma with a marked variation in cell types and an abundance of mitotic figures.

Postoperatively there was no voluntary movement of his left upper arm or leg. Two weeks after surgery the left leg was paralyzed and spastic. A moderate weakness was present in his left shoulder and upper arm. A left extensor plantar response (Babinski's sign) was present. There were no sensory deficits. The patient then received supervoltage radiation therapy.

Paralysis of his left leg continued, but the patient could walk with a circumducting gait. He experienced occasional simple partial seizures, beginning in the left hand. Otherwise, he did well for the next 6 months, at which point increasing spastic weakness in his left arm developed. With the development of increased intracranial pressure, the patient became obtunded and developed papilledema. He died 2 days later.

The location of disease in this case was clear from the neurologic deficits and was confirmed by imaging studies. The history suggested a rapidly growing, non–space-occupying tumor such as a glioblastoma. Marked weakness in the lower leg suggested a localization in the motor cortex down in the interhemispheric fissure, where the tumor was found. The persistent paralysis of the left leg after surgery likewise corresponded to the area of greatest ablation.

The initial simple partial seizures involving the left shoulder correspond to the shoulder area relatively high on the precentral gyrus, close to the area of tumor involvement. In general, partial seizures do not originate from dysfunctional cortical areas but from adjacent cortical areas of partial damage or of altered function. Thus, although weakness was greatest in the leg, seizures originated from the shoulder or hand areas.

The purpose of surgery in this case was to confirm the preoperative impression of an intrinsic tumor and to obtain a histologic diagnosis of the tumor. As much of the tumor mass as possible was removed. This reduced the tumor's pressure on the surviving, relatively normal cortical areas within the closed cranial cavity to preserve their function.

Glioblastomas are highly malignant tumors that usually lack clearly defined borders. Even though some enucleation may be performed as in this case, a surgical cure is virtually impossible. Tumor cells have already invaded apparently normal areas of the white matter and cortex. The late effects reflect tumor regrowth, the invasion of other areas, and the increased pressure effects of the tumor.

Tumors of the Central Nervous System

Most tumors of brain cells are of glial cell origin as was the glioblastoma described in the case history. Glial tumors make up about half of all intercranial tumors. There is no clear line between tumor and healthy brain.

In contrast to the glioblastoma just discussed, astrocytomas grow slowly and are more amenable to surgery and radiotherapy. Survival for 5 and 10 years is common. Astrocytomas become space occupying and increase intercranial pressure late in their course.

Tumors of the coverings of the brain, *meningiomas*, are common. Because they are not of the brain itself, meningiomas are well encapsulated and occupy space fairly early in their course. Because they occupy space, these tumors cause increased intercranial pressure and its symptoms (papilledema, nausea and vomiting, headache, and possible herniation). They often can be totally excised and rarely metastasize.

Metastatic tumors from neoplasms of other organs, particularly the lung, are similarly encapsulated, occupy space, and can be removed. They may, however, be multiple. Both meningiomas and metastatic tumors are uncommon before age 50.

Tumors of the pituitary (see Fig. 4-20) are also common. In addition to causing disturbed pituitary function, these tumors often press on the base of the brain in the region of the optic chiasm; bitemporal hemianopsia results. Tumors of the pituitary can be treated by surgery and radiotherapy.

POST-TEST

1. Where is sound perceived? Where is it heard as language?

2. Where is pain perceived? Localized? What methods are available to lessen pain?

3. Where do the fine motor movements of the fingers begin? What structures must be intact for a hand grasp to occur?

4. What region of the cerebrum is implicated in personality change?

5. What is the function of the corpus callosum? What problems do you think its destruction would cause?

6. Draw a diagram of the circle of Willis.

7. What are the major symptoms of a subarachnoid hemorrhage?

8. How large an area does the corticospinal tract occupy in the internal capsule as compared with the area of the precentral gyrus?

9. What is the sequence of signs presented by an extradural hematoma?

10. What major functional areas of the cerebrum are supplied by the left middle cerebral artery?

CASE HISTORIES

1. A left-handed 8-year-old was hit in the left side of the head by a baseball. He fell to the ground and was found unconscious. He regained consciousness but was very groggy and did not answer questions. He is taken to a small, nearby emergency department. When plain skull films show a depressed fracture in the temporal-parietal-coronal suture area, he is transferred to a trauma center. On admission, he is conscious but responds incoherently to questions. Both pupils reacted briskly to light.

2. A 28-year-old research worker had a massive seizure last night. He is presently without any signs of disease. He remembers waking up and feeling his arm and face moving and then blacking out. He and his wife have just returned from a cross country 2-day bus trip during which they got very little sleep. His wife describes the attack as follows: "His right arm started twitching, which woke me up; when I turned on the light, his face was also twitching. Pretty soon his right leg was twitching as well. The whole thing lasted one-half hour. He wouldn't answer me until he woke up 3 hours later." He has had a number of episodes of twitching of

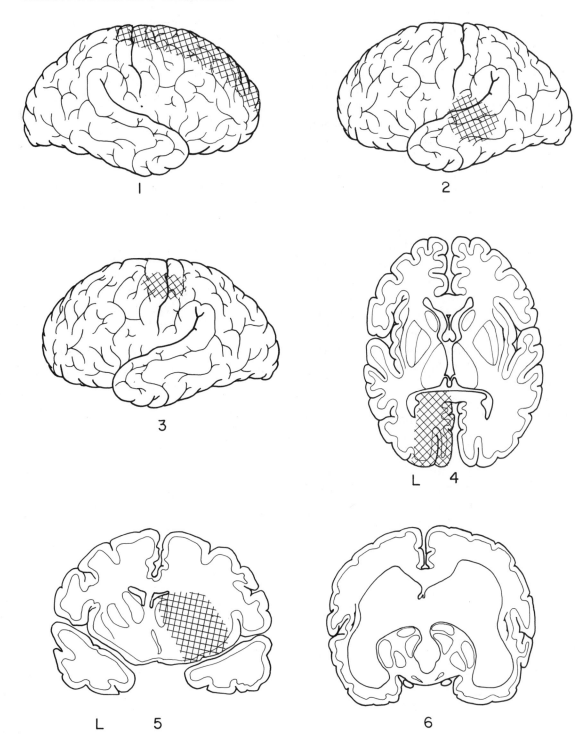

LESION DIAGRAMS: CEREBRUM

the right side of his face or right face and right arm over the last 4 years. He noticed that it was hard to think after these twitching attacks.

3. Ms. J. J. is 57 years old and burned her left hand last week. After the burn was dressed, the emergency room physician suggested she seek further medical advice. She has episodes of clumsiness of her left hand since she had a mastectomy last year. On examination, she is alert and cooperative but has not buttoned her left shirt cuff or put polish on the fingernails of her left hand. She cannot accurately localize pinprick or touch on her left hand and arm. She cannot recognize a dime when it is placed on her left hand or identify which number is drawn on her left hand. All other examinations were negative except for a left Babinski's response.

4. G. J., a 39-year-old male, has had a numb feeling in his left leg for some months. The numbness seems to be getting worse. The leg is strong, and reflexes are normal. He can perceive pinprick but cannot localize it. All other sensations are much more di-

minished on the left leg compared with the right.

5. J. K., a 79-year-old male, had a colon carcinoma removed 18 months ago. He now suffers from a deep burning pain in his right pelvis. A bone scan shows multiple metastases to the pelvis and long bones. Aspirin controlled the pain at first, but now he needs codeine every 3 hours. What are the therapeutic options?

6. J. S., a 38-year-old female, has had a strange feeling of numbness in her left side and leg that has gradually gotten worse in the last few months. She has now lost pinprick sensation on the entire left side below the breast. Babinski's response on the right is positive. All other physical findings are negative.

7. G. Q., a 33-year-old plumber, has had shooting pains down the outside of the right leg that last 5 to 10 minutes and occur two or three times a week, particularly in the evenings. The fear of another attack often keeps him awake. Demerol has very little effect on the pain. If all other signs are negative, what course do you advise? If the right ankle jerk is weak, what course do you advise?

6

Control of Movement

At first thought, movement is easy enough to describe: I reach out and pick up a pencil. But is it so simple? First, I must be sitting upright, not falling to one side. Second, I must be able to adjust my posture to counterbalance the weight of my extended arm. Third, I extend my arm with a smooth, fluid movement directly toward the pencil. Last, I oppose my thumb and forefinger to capture the pencil. I have used 50 to 60 different muscles to do this apparently simple task. Perhaps the best way to describe or define movement is as a series of postures with fine limb motion appended.

For many years movement was described by the anatomic structures thought to be responsible. The *pyramidal* tract (named for the pyramids in the medulla, see Fig. 4-7)—today called the *corticospinal* tract—was thought to be the route of all conscious commands. Hence, the phrase *pyramidal system* referred to the corticospinal pathway for initiation and control of voluntary movement.

All other pathways and movements were formerly lumped into the *extrapy-*

ramidal system. When muscle spindles were discovered, some authors suggested that the pyramidal system innervated [α] motor neurons, while the extrapyramidal system innervated γ motor neurons. It is now clear that such a view is, unfortunately, much too simple. Because the terms pyramidal and extrapyramidal have so many varying connotations, I propose to use them no further. The terms are included here because they were once widely used and you should know of their existence.

MOTOR-SENSORY INTEGRATION

All parts of the nervous system that participate in voluntary motor activity belong to the *motor system*. The motor system certainly includes such structures as the premotor areas, the precentral gyri, the corticospinal tracts, the anterior horns, and the peripheral nerves and muscles discussed in Chapter 2. It includes many more structures we will discuss in this chapter.

We should keep in mind that a motor system without information on where it is and where it is going is about as useful as a blind person driving a large truck at high speed. The motor system generates motor commands that are modulated both by sensory input and by a sense of purpose. This modulation occurs at a number of levels in the nervous system. As we have already discussed, these structures exist on both sides of the neuroaxis and, to keep confusion to a minimum, I will discuss only one side. The structures on the other side of the neuroaxis act similarly. Five major levels of motor-sensory integration are:

Frontal lobe-parietal lobe
Basal ganglia-thalamus
Red nucleus-anterior cerebellum
Vestibular nucleus-labyrinth
Anterior-posterior horns of spinal cord

All these levels function harmoniously in an intact nervous system. The great challenge is to tease function from a damaged brain. To do so, the capabilities of each level must be understood. Let's start at the spinal cord and work our way up the neuroaxis.

Anterior-Posterior Horns

We have already discussed spinal reflexes that use only one or two segments of the spinal cord. Certainly the stretch reflex is the simplest example of motor-sensory integration. More extensive reflexes spread to the opposite side in the cord, such as the crossed extensor reflex response to pain. The spinal cord of four-legged animals is capable of more extensive motor integration. Scratching a moving target, such as a flea, and alternating gait are examples. In humans, chewing gum may be an example of a reflexive response. The grasp reflex, flexing the fingers without thumb motion, is a complex, multisegment reflex.

Vestibular Nuclei-Labyrinth

The labyrinth of the inner ear, including the semicircular canals, provides information on the body's position in space to the vestibular nucleus and to the midline cerebellum (Fig. 6-1). The midline cerebellum feeds information back to vestibular nuclei. Vestibular nuclei also receive input from the stretch receptors in the neck. Two new types of sensory information are added at this level: position of the head in space and position of the head in relation to the body. Both are very important in maintaining posture. A patient with Ménière's disease gets false information from the labyrinth and usually ends up falling.

F I G U R E 6-1
The major structures of the motor system and the specific major inputs and outputs of the vestibular nuclei. The brain stem and cerebellum are hemisected up to the level of the midbrain.

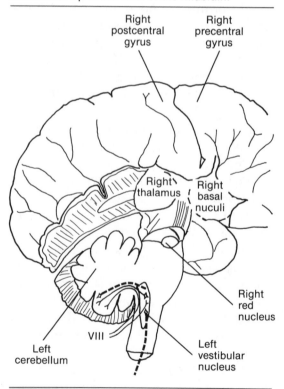

The *vestibulospinal tract* descends in the anterior column of the spinal cord. In general, extensor reflexes are facilitated and flexor reflexes are inhibited by vestibulospinal activity. Proximal muscles are more affected than are distal muscles. Axons of the vestibulospinal tract terminate primarily on γ motor neurons. The spasticity of a lateral spinal cord lesion may be the result of unopposed vestibulospinal tract activity.

Red Nucleus-Anterior Cerebellum

The anterior cerebellum receives the ipsilateral spinocerebellar tracts (Fig. 6-2). The left side of the cerebellum relates to the left side of the body. Fibers leave the left cerebellum by way of the superior cerebellar peduncle, cross the midline, and enter the right red nucleus. The right red nucleus relates in turn to the left side of the body.

F I G U R E 6-2
The major connections of the red nucleus-anterior cerebellum complex.

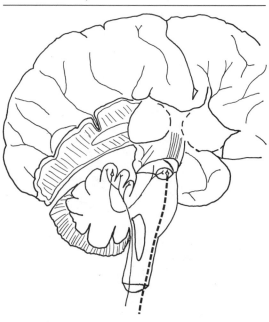

F I G U R E 6-3
The major connections of the basal nuclei-thalamus complex.

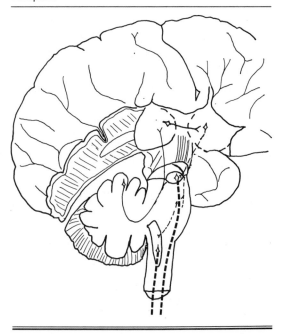

The *rubrospinal tract* crosses the neuroaxis soon after emerging from the red nucleus. This tract contains fibers that both facilitate flexor motor neurons and inhibit extensor motor neurons. Proximal muscles are heavily influenced, but this tract also influences distal muscles. The rubrospinal tract heavily influences both γ and α motor neuron activity.

Basal Ganglia-Thalamus

The thalamus receives all the direct sensory tracts. These include the spinothalamic tract and the posterior columns-medial lemniscus system. The right thalamus relates to the left side of the body. The thalamus also receives much of the outflow from the contralateral cerebellum (Fig. 6-3).

The majority of the outflow from the basal ganglia is to the thalamus for relay to the precentral and postcentral gyri.

There are descending connections from the basal ganglia to the red nucleus and probably to the vestibular nucleus, but no major direct connections continue to the spinal cord. The basal ganglia receive the major outflow of the premotor frontal lobe cortex and some outflow from the thalamus.

Frontal-Parietal Lobes

Each parietal lobe, particularly the postcentral gyrus, receives the major sensory tracts relayed by the thalamus (Fig. 6-4). Motor-sensory and proprioceptive information from the cerebellum and basal ganglia, also relayed by the thalamus, reaches both frontal and parietal lobes.

Corticospinal and *corticobulbar* tracts rise in the precentral gyrus, in the premotor area, and in many other parts of the cerebrum, including the postcentral gyrus. From this large area the tracts converge, pass through the internal capsule, and descend through the cerebral peduncle of the midbrain. The corticobulbar tracts innervate the cranial nerve motor nuclei and, through synapses in the pons, the cerebellum. The corticospinal tracts cross the neuroaxis in the low medulla. The tracts travel in the lateral columns of the spinal cord with almost half of the fibers ending in the cervical segments.

There are two types of output from the frontal lobe; each type is the result of conscious processes. One type is the direct corticospinal output (Fig. 6-4). A supine person raising a finger is an example. This direct type of motor outflow is most apparent in hand and facial movements and corresponds to their huge representation on the precentral gyrus.

The second type of frontal lobe motor output involves an idea of a more complex movement. One such idea could be to swing at an inside curve ball

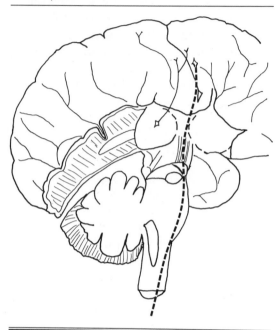

F I G U R E 6-4
The thalamocortical projections and the corticospinal tract.

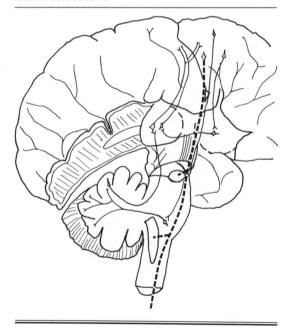

F I G U R E 6-5
The feedback circuit between the cerebral cortex and the basal nuclei-thalamus complex and the lateral cerebellum.

when you are at bat. The idea is sent from the premotor area to the basal ganglia and cerebellum (Fig. 6-5). There the idea is amplified, and more specific instructions are generated. These much more specific instructions are returned to the frontal lobe (via the thalamus) for implementation and transmission via the corticospinal tract. Some of these amplified instructions are undoubtedly sent to the red and vestibular nuclei for execution. These instructions presumably involve postural changes.

STIMULATION OF MOTOR CORTEX

Precentral gyrus stimulation results in contraction of muscle groups, but never in purposeful movements. There is a very short delay between stimulation and muscle movement. Neurons stimulating synergistic muscles are arranged in columns separated from the columns of neurons controlling antagonistic muscles.

In contrast, when regions of the premotor area are stimulated, more integrated movements—such as turning the head and eyes—are elicited. There is a considerable delay between cortical stimulation and the complex movement. Enough time elapses to activate the premotor-basal ganglia-thalamus and the premotor-cerebellum-thalamus circuits back to the precentral gyrus.

ABLATION

Studying the motor capability of the severed neuroaxis has contributed greatly to our understanding of the ability of the individual levels of motor-sensory integration to act independently. A transverse section of the nervous system creates two parts, one with connections to the precentral gyrus and one without connections to the precentral gyrus. We will discuss the function of the part without connections to the precentral gyrus but with connections to anterior horn cells. In Chapter 3 we discussed the severed spinal cord and the gradual return of spinal reflexes. We continue to underestimate the integrative ability of the spinal cord.

Decerebrate rigidity, an immediate extensor rigidity, develops when the neuroaxis is severed in the midbrain region (Fig. 6-6). The pons, medulla, and spinal cord remain functional. Tentorial herniation (see Fig. 4-3) is a frequent cause of decerebrate rigidity. Both extensors and flexors are active, and any attempt to move the limb meets with immediate resistance. The vestibular nuclei are the source of this extensor tone; if they also are destroyed, the rigidity disappears. Further, most of this extensor tone is

F I G U R E 6-6
Decerebrate rigidity. (After Fulton, J. F.: *A Textbook of Physiology*. Philadelphia, W. B. Saunders Co., 1955.)

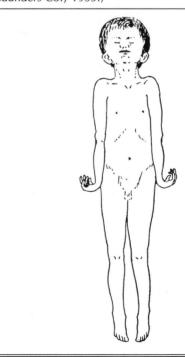

dependent on intact posterior roots, strongly implicating the γ system.

Decorticate rigidity results from a dysfunction just above the red nucleus and gives a very different picture (Fig. 6-7). In humans, the arms are flexed and are easily influenced by head-on-neck reflexes. The arm extends on the side the head is turned toward.

When only the cerebral cortex is damaged, the basal nuclei and thalamus are left intact. Dogs and cats with damage to the cerebral cortex only can run, balance, and, in fact, do practically everything a blind animal can do with the exception of placing their feet accurately. Remember, these animals would be blind because they have also lost the visual cortex. While the descending motor pathways from the basal ganglia are not clear, their presence adds greatly to

motor control. Such extensive lesions of the cerebral cortex alone are rare, or are still unrecognized in humans.

Ablation of small parts of a precentral gyrus deprives patients of specific movements, such as flexing and extending the third finger. The finger can, however, participate in more complex movements such as grasp.

When the corticospinal tracts alone are severed, either in the midbrain or the medulla, there is an initial paralysis without spasticity. In dogs and cats, almost all motion returns except finer movements of the forepaw. In monkeys, recovery takes longer. Axial and postural movement, such as walking, is intact but fine hand movements, such as grasping, do not return. Reports of similar human lesions are sparse.

DEVELOPMENTAL-PHYLOGENETIC CLUES

Human corticospinal tracts are unmyelinated at birth, and myelination is not complete until age 20 to 25 months. Tracking the development of motor activity in human infants gives us many clues about the ability of parts of the nervous system to function without the corticospinal tracts. At birth, infants can breathe, cry, and suckle. By 6 months they can roll over; brain stem motor centers are now functioning. Further brain stem function is evident when the 6- to 12-month-old child learns to crawl. Increasing skill demonstrates increasing cerebral guidance. Hand placement is poorly coordinated, and hand function is limited to the spinal reflex, grasp.

By 18 months—and often by 10 to 12 months—a child can pull itself upright and toddle around as the corticospinal tracts are fairly well myelinated. Further motor development includes running, fine control of balance, coordination,

F I G U R E 6-7
Decorticate rigidity. (After Fulton, J. F.: *A Textbook of Physiology.* Philadelphia, W. B. Saunders Co., 1955.)

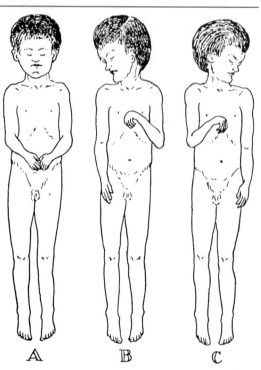

A   B   C

and fine hand movements. These are rarely completed before 6 to 8 years of age.

Increased motor skills and central nervous system (CNS) complexities are found in the ascending orders of vertebrates. Both provide clues on the ability of each of the sensory-motor levels already discussed to act independently. Swimming, in a fish, is usually done in one of three speeds and is carried out largely as a spinal cord reflex. The brain stem keeps the fish upright and directs it toward food and mates and away from danger.

The frog hops, the salamander waddles; both actions are largely spinal reflexes with balance provided by brain stem nuclei. It is the cerebellum that is much larger in these animals. Reptiles and lower mammals exhibit some independent activity in their individual limbs, but not much.

Mammals show an increasing ability to use their limbs independently. Humans and the great apes show the greatest agility and have the largest frontal lobes and basal nuclei.

MOVEMENT DISORDERS

Coordinated movement is very important to our everyday life. Any change in our ability to move is quickly noticed, and we seek help. There is a wide variety of movement disorders; some of the more common ones follow.

Paralysis and *paresis* (weakness) are the most common movement problems. Upper and lower motor neuron lesions have already been described. If the lesion is in the upper motor neurons, possibilities for retraining exist; other intact descending pathways are used to activate anterior horn cells.

Precentral gyrus lesions usually paralyze only part of the body. Lesions of the entire precentral gyrus are unusual because of its length. Lesions of the internal capsule cause paralysis of contralateral face, arm, and leg. Lesions of the cerebral peduncle of the midbrain paralyze the contralateral face, arm, leg, and ipsilateral cranial nerve III. Lesions of the medulla and upper cervical cord cause arm and leg paralysis. Lesions in the lateral thoracic cord result in ipsilateral leg paralysis.

Spasticity is the next most common movement disorder. It is often combined with paralysis or paresis but can occur without weakness. Spasticity defines an active or passive movement that is supple for short or slow movements but meets resistance for longer or rapid movements. Most patients show a spastic extensor leg and a spastic flexed and pronated arm. The tract (or perhaps the nucleus) responsible for spasticity is not clear. The few humans with pure corticospinal tract lesions in either the midbrain or the medulla have not shown spasticity.

Lesions causing spasticity and paralysis are large ones. Plugging one middle cerebral artery destroys a large area of the frontal and parietal lobes and produces a spastic paralysis of the face and hand..

A lesion in the internal capsule causes a spastic hemiparesis (face, arm, and leg). Rising direct sensory tracts, as well as returning instructions from the cerebellum and basal nuclei, are interrupted. In addition to the corticospinal tract, tracts descending to the brain stem are compromised.

Common brain stem lesions involving one or both corticospinal tracts usually cause only limited spasticity, perhaps because the corticospinal tracts are isolated from other descending motor systems in the anterior brain stem.

When the lateral columns of the spinal cord are damaged, intense spasticity is present. The vestibular nuclei are important in facilitating spasticity because their destruction alleviates the condition.

Rigidity is another abnormal activity adversely affecting movement. Rigidity differs from spasticity by its constant muscle activity, even in the resting position. The resistance to both active and passive movement is immediate and progressive. Rigidity is often described as lead-pipe rigidity; it has the malleable quality of twisting a lead pipe or a piece of thick taffy. A very common finding in Parkinson's disease, rigidity makes all movement very difficult. It originates in the basal ganglia.

Resting tremors are caused by dysfunction in the basal ganglia-thalamus complex. They can frequently be treated by stereotactic surgery that destroys part of the feedback circuit between the frontal lobe, basal ganglia, thalamus, and precentral gyrus (Fig. 6-5). These tremors disappear during sleep. The pill-rolling tremor of the hands seen in Parkinsonian patients is typical of resting tremors. Similar symptoms are caused by the side effects of a number of common psychotropic drugs.

Intention tremors occur during movement and have their origin in the cerebellum. The patient's hand is steady at rest. As the hand moves toward the examiner's finger, the tremor gets worse. When the patient's hand reaches that of the examiner, the tremor ends. Tumors of the cerebellum or chronic alcoholism produce intention tremors.

Involuntary movements are much grosser movements than tremors. They can have their origin either as a localized seizure in one frontal lobe or as abnormal activity in the basal ganglia. Localized seizures are usually completely purposeless movements and can be diagnosed by electroencephalography

(EEG) or by observation of the seizure as it spreads through the body.

Involuntary movements caused by pathology in the basal ganglia include *choreiform* movements. They are abrupt and jerky and begin when the patient is in a resting posture. The movements can occur frequently. *Athetosis* describes an almost constant, sinuous movement of the face, hands, or both and the arms. Patients can move their arms or hands, but it is almost impossible for them to maintain any posture. *Torsion dystonia* refers to a movement disorder that results in an abnormal posture lasting for days or weeks. Ultimately there can be deformity of the spine.

Loss of *associated movements*, such as swinging the arms during walking, occurs in basal ganglia disorders. Patients who take short, shuffling steps and keep their arms hanging at their sides are telegraphing a disturbance of the basal ganglia.

Abnormal reflexes are those that are normally suppressed but become evident because of a disease process. Babinski's sign is an example. The infantile response, a spinal reflex, is suppressed by the corticospinal tract at about 2 years of age. Its appearance later in life is a sure sign of corticospinal tract dysfunction. Similarly, the grasp reflex of the hand and pursing the lips, as in sucking, are reflexes that are suppressed by the frontal lobe and appear when frontal lobe dysfunction occurs.

Cerebral palsy describes a wide group of movement disorders present at, or soon after, birth. Only the most severe are immediately apparent. The majority of cases show slow development. The full extent of the disability may not be apparent for 3 to 6 years. Pathology may occur in the cortex, basal nuclei, or cerebellum to give spasticity, athetosis, or ataxia, respectively. Very often there are mixtures of these symptoms in the patient. Intensive physical, occupational, and speech therapy can often be of great assistance in helping these patients lead useful and independent lives.

Parkinson's disease, primarily an affliction of older persons, results in rigidity, tremor, and an inability to begin movements (akinesia). The cause of the disease is unknown, but it is very incapacitating. Patients sit for hours without moving except for the pill-rolling tremor. The tremor has been treated by lesions surgically placed in the thalamus. The greatest advance in treatment came with the introduction of *dopa*, (see Chapter 8), a neurotransmitter. While dopa is not a panacea, it reduces the rigidity and akinesia remarkably.

TYPES OF MOTOR CONTROL

To help you comprehend function and dysfunction in the motor system, I have devised three ways of categorizing movement: A. routes to the spinal cord; B. commands controlling movement; and C. levels of complexity of movement. These categories overlap, but how is not yet clear.

A. Routes to the Spinal Cord

Human postural patterns and limb movements begin with an idea in the brain. Three major descending systems carry motor commands, for implementation of the idea, to the anterior horn cells of the spinal cord:

A1. *Vestibular outflow* controls axial movements. This outflow is influenced by the body's position in space, by the relation of the head to the neck, and by motor commands from the cerebral cortex. This system determines posture, whether sitting, standing, or hanging by the knees.

A2. *Red nucleus outflow* adds the ability to use the limbs independently, particularly the arms. This outflow is modulated by the position of the limbs in relation to the body and by motor commands from the cerebral cortex.

A3. *Cerebral cortical outflow* enables the manipulation of the forearm and hand in highly specific tasks.

B. Commands Controlling Movement

Body movements differ widely from one other. Five different responses to movement commands can be described (with examples given):

B1. *Response to direct command*—to contract 14 motor units of the right adductor pollicis and hold a pencil.

B2. *Facilitation of existing reflexes*—to reach for and grasp a piece of candy (as a 2-year-old learns how to do).

B3. *Inhibition of existing reflexes*—to inhibit the positive supporting reflex of the right leg so that the right leg flexors can raise the leg off the ground and reach the next step.

B4. *Maintenance of posture*—to remain sitting upright in a car turning a corner.

B5. *Movement from posture to posture*—to go from lying on your back to sitting upright.

C. Movement Complexity

Different levels of complexity coexist to establish movement and posture:

C1. *Instinctive movements* include four-legged walking in a dog or cat or crawling in humans. Most of the neural connections for instinctive movements and postures are organized at either a spinal cord or low brain-stem level. They need little more than a single descending command to activate them.

C2. *Learned movements and postures* are those used or practiced for many years. Playing musical chords with the left hand is an example. These movements are difficult to learn but gradually become easier and easier until they need very little thought. Upright walking may well belong in this category. (An analogy might be to that of programming a computer; it is difficult to do, but once the program is written, single commands cause lots to happen.)

C3. *New learned movements* are difficult and require concentration. For myself, learning to thread a needle was hard, and because I don't do it frequently, it remains a complex motor task. These motions probably require the full attention of both precentral and postcentral gyri. Each part of every submovement must be checked, usually by visual feed-

back. Only the basic posture (e.g., sitting up) can be set in advance. When repeated often enough, however, these can become learned movements.

One could use this classification to diagram a type C3 movement, threading a needle (Fig. 6-8). For example, movement begins with type A3 cerebral outflow activating type B1 commands to the hand, type B2 commands to the arm by type A1 outflow, and type B4 commands by type A2 outflow to the rest of the body.

FIGURE 6-8
Possible pathways linking a cerebral command to muscle movement.

C3 COMMAND (THREAD NEEDLE)

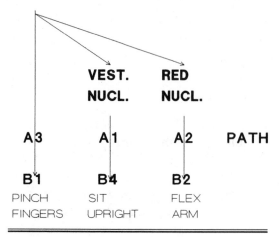

VEST. NUCL.	RED NUCL.

A3	A1	A2	PATH
B1	B4	B2	
PINCH FINGERS	SIT UPRIGHT	FLEX ARM	

POST-TEST

1. Construct diagrams similar to Figure 6-8 for the following movements:
   a. Controlling a sewing machine with a foot-activated control.
   b. Controlling the speed of a car with the gas pedal.
   c. Crawling along a narrow plank.
   d. Munching potato chips.

2. Gather all the information in this chapter about each major sensory-motor integration center onto a block diagram. Pair the sensory-motor levels vertically. Keep the sensory tracts and centers on the left and the motor centers and tracts on the right. You may find that coloring in copies of this diagram helps you answer the questions that follow.

3. What types of commands do you expect the vestibular system to carry out?

4. What types of movement do you expect the red nuclei to participate in?

5. How do you picture the cerebral cortex's involvement in
   a. Walking.
   b. Throwing a baseball.

   c. Threading a needle.

   d. Learning to print with the non-dominant hand.

6. Contrast the dysfunction you would expect after a stroke in the lower right precentral gyrus or in the right internal capsule.

7. Be prepared to demonstrate both a resting tremor and an intention tremor.

8. What descending pathways do you think a hemiplegic patient uses when walking with the circumducting gait that is characteristic of these patients?

9. What pathways are stimulated when a child is placed prone on a giant floppy ball and rolled around? When a infant is placed supine in a crib?

10. What movement deficit would you expect if only the postcentral gyrus were destroyed?

11. What is the role of each level of the motor system in the following movements?

   a. A sailor's upright posture while the ship is listing to the right and when the ship is rolling from right to left.

   b. A fireman climbing a ladder versus a 6-year-old child learning to climb a ladder.

   c. Learning to type versus typing after many years of continuous practice.

CASE HISTORIES

1. (Case courtesy of Peggy Stewart, O.T.R., Ph.D., University of Illinois College of Allied Health Sciences, Chicago):

A 46-year-old male, admitted to the hospital for neurologic work-up, was referred to occupational therapy. The neurosurgeon requested OT to "evaluate everything; so far we have found nothing abnormal in our tests. Try to give us some clue as to what is going on."

Results of the OT evaluations were normal ROM and MMT; normal sensation including pinprick, one and two point discrimination, stereognosis, and touch; normal mental functions of oriented times 3, long term memory, and basic mathematics. Some minor problems were noted in screening tests for figure-ground discrimination, spatial orientation, and kinesthesia.

A modified post-rotary nystagmus test was administered with the patient seated in a wheelchair and the chair rotated three revolutions. The patient responded to this with all color draining form his face, a weak but rapid pulse, and rapid, shallow respiration. A rapid nystagmus response was noted. The patient held his head and assumed a slumped posture.

The OT, aware of the crisis response, prepared to call a code blue, however, the reaction slowly decreased over 15 minutes with the patient then demonstrating normal vital functions. Questioning the patient regarding this reaction he stated, "I don't understand this; as a kid I could ride merry-go-rounds and roller-coasters with the best of them."

Upon reporting the patient's response to the physician, it was suggested that an abnormality existed in the 8th cranial nerve system. Further testing revealed a small acoustic neuroma which was surgically removed. OT treated the patient postoperatively and found the abnormalities

The following outlines of the lateral surface of the cerebrum show areas of increased blood flow associated with particular movements. Blood flow increased because both excitatory and inhibitory neuronal activity increased. What structures are included in each area? What are each of these structures contributing to the movement? (Traced from the work of Lassen, N., Ingar, D., and Skinhei, E. *Arch Neurol,* 33:523, 1976.)

ACTIVE AREAS DURING MOVEMENT

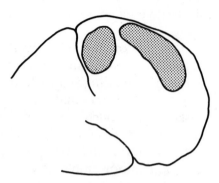

Hand squeezing ball

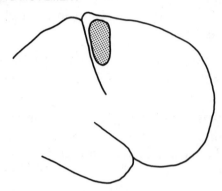

"Squeezing" ball with arm anesthetized

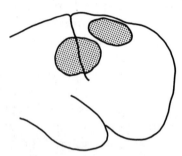

Shape discrimination with hand (active finger movement)

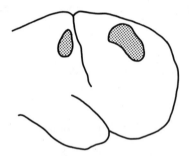

Shape discrimination (passive finger movement)

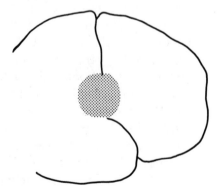

Shape discrimination with mouth and tongue

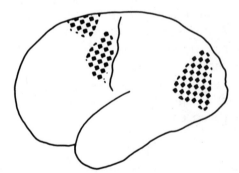

Eyes following swinging ping-pong ball

in visual-perceptual-motor function were more involved than the initial screening suggested. However, after interviewing the patient and his wife it was clear these deficits were present for many years and were not secondary to the surgical procedure. An outpatient treatment program was initiated to develop those functions. He made rapid improvement over a 4-week period and reported for the first time in 20 years he had done the bookkeeping for his small trucking business. He said, "I always thought I was dumb since I couldn't manage the books. Now I know it was a physical problem that prevented me from putting the numbers in the right columns.

2. (Case courtesy of Peggy Stewart, O.T.R., Ph.D., University of Illinois College of Allied Health Sciences, Chicago):

     A 17-year-old male was admitted to the hospital with a fracture-dislocation of the T6 vertebrae sustained in a fall. He was placed on a striker frame for 4 weeks. Rehabilitation was initiated at bedside and progressed to a full program in the department within 1 week after traction was discontinued. The rehab program was uneventful with the patient making rapid gains in wheelchair motility, upper extremity strength, and self-care activities. One complication was reported by the physical therapist. This was hyperreflexia of the lower extremities. The hyperreflexia was a problem for application of long leg braces and attempts to ambulate in the parallel bars. The PT suggested that medication to reduce the reflexia should be considered.

     Later that day, the OT asked the patient about this. He reported, "Yes, when I try to get up and walk in PT my legs just stick straight out. It also happens sometimes when I am in my room."

     Working that afternoon together, they found that a knee-jerk reflex was stimulated if the patient rotated his shoulders to the right, then elevated the left shoulder and depressed the right. The reflex was sustained as long as the position was maintained and subsided as soon as the position was released. Reversing the direction of the position had no effect on the reflex. With this knowledge the patient began training in transfer techniques for bed and bathtub using the reflex to raise the legs. Also the problem in PT was eliminated by reversing the hand position to the right on parallel bars and left on the wheelchair armrest. Using this approach, medication was avoided since it is often unsuccessful and when it does work it affects reflexes at all levels not just those below the level of injury.

3. A 47-year-old salesman has held many different jobs, has married three times, and describes himself as a social drinker. He has an unsteady gait, walks with his feet wide apart and watches his feet. Muscle strength is intact; so are pinprick and vibration sense. There is no resting tremor. As he moves his finger toward the examiner a course side to side tremor develops which fades as his finger reaches the examiner. Heel to shin testing is similarly ataxic. Optic disk is normal. MRI scan of posterior fossa is read as normal with perhaps a slight enlargement of IV ventrical.

4. A 32-year-old female beautician had several spells 16 months ago which began on the left side of the face; the twitching has since spread to the shoulder, hand, and foot. She noticed a little tingling in the tongue

and face after these attacks. She was placed on Dilantin and had no further attacks. Two weeks ago the patient had a very similar seizure and afterward she noticed her arm was weak. She has been having increasingly severe headaches lately, often taking eight to ten aspirin a day to relieve them.

Upon examination she shows weakness of her left face and arm with increased reflexes on the left side. There were no sensory disturbances.

Where is the pathology? Why do you place it there? What is the most likely cause of the seizures 16 months ago? What is the most likely cause of the headaches? What would be reasonable diagnostic studies? Why?

5. Emily J. is a 52-year-old single charge nurse who has had increasing difficulty in the last year or so "getting along" with the nurses, doctors, and patients on her unit. Previously, she had been well liked, very tidy, and efficient. Now she is careless about her appearance and her office is a mess; she can't find anything and the shift nurses are keeping duplicate records. She walks with a shuffling gait and has difficulty turning.

Upon examination she has brisk reflexes on the right and both right and left toes are extensor. Voluntary strength is somewhat diminished on the right side. Grasp and suck reflexes are easily elicited.

Where is the lesion? Speculate on pathology and prognosis.

7

Language

Although language defies accurate definition, it includes the mental ability to relate objects seen, heard, or felt with spoken words and the ability to translate these objects into speech or writing. No matter which sense (vision, hearing, touch, smell, or taste) we use to receive the message of fresh popcorn, we can make the same judgment about the message: Eat it! As important, language involves the ability to think symbolically about concepts much more abstract than popcorn.

The spoken word "cross" evokes the same connotations as does a cross seen or felt. You can draw a cross in response to the spoken word "cross." To speak the word "cross" either when shown a picture of a cross or when you have had a cross drawn on the palm of your hand are other examples of your ability to carry a symbolic idea across sensory (receptive) and motor (expressive) modalities. We convert each of these inputs into a *language code,* compare them with our experience, and then express this language code by a variety of means. This discussion will concentrate on right-handed persons with a dominant

left hemisphere and will consider left-handedness later.

DYSPHASIAS

The partial loss of language function, particularly the loss of a single language function such as speech, is known as *dysphasia.* The cerebral regions for the various receptive, expressive, and cognitive functions of language are scattered throughout the dominant hemisphere. Small- to medium-sized lesions are more likely to impair a single language function severely than to impair all language functions partially. Identifying any remaining language functions and helping dysphasic patients to use these functions greatly improve the quality of their lives.

Aphasia is the total inability to deal with language. It is frequently used, unfortunately, to describe diminished language ability. This is particularly true with spoken language. Aphasia evokes many emotional connotations just as the word "cancer" does. For this reason it is best avoided, especially when describing partial language deficits.

Because so much of our interpersonal communication is based on speech, the ability to receive and produce spoken language is usually tested first: "Good morning, feeling great today?" On reflection, we do not expect a person who is deaf or who does not speak English to respond. A 4-month-old child is hardly aphasic. We should tailor our expectations to the circumstances.

There are a number of common dysphasias, each an important clinical problem. Dysphasias can be subdivided into expressive, receptive, or cognitive dysphasias. Each gives us a clue to the function of the cortical areas involved in language. By using the term dysphasia rather than the older term aphasia, I hope you will remember that affected patients retain some language functions. They need help in communicating effectively.

Expressive Dysphasias

Expressive dysphasia involves the inability to communicate ideas, either by the spoken or written words. Patients know what they want to express. The basic muscles needed are intact. The person cannot transform the language code of what they wish to express into a motor idea that activates the appropriate muscles.

Handwriting apraxia, an inability to form letters, arises with lesions of the dominant premotor cortex. The right hand can only move clumsily. The patient cannot convert an idea (language code) into written or printed language and cannot use a typewriter. Very clever pointing devices, attached to an apraxic patient's head, allow use of a computer to output language.

Patients with *Broca's dysphasia* cannot speak or produce the appropriate words only with great difficulty. Facial muscles and vocal cords are intact. These patients clearly comprehend spoken language and can follow serial commands, such as "place your left hand to your nose and then to your left ear." They know what they wish to say and can write it, but they cannot speak what is on their mind.

The area affected in Broca's dysphasia is the inferior premotor cortex, also called Broca's area (Fig. 7-1). This area converts language code into motor commands for syllables and is an extension of the premotor cortex where motor ideas begin. As the precentral gyrus is intact, patients can control their facial muscles and can make some sounds but not syllables. A few simple, commonly used words such as "no" are often preserved in patients with severe lesions of Broca's area. Presumably there is enough capacity in the precentral gyrus to generate these simple words.

Patients with Broca's dysphasia may have to communicate by waving a hand or foot, blinking their eyes, or by pointing to an appropriate object. Patients decide the message they wish to convey and then find a way to transmit the idea. Gestures are an effective means of communication for impaired and non-impaired individuals alike (e.g., thumbs up, thumbs down or "OK" sign). Boards with pictures of important objects or actions can greatly help patients communicate with the caregiver.

Many patients with Broca's dysphasia retain the ability to sing. You may feel self-conscious singing "Happy Birthday," but they will usually join in. Therapies have been developed to help these patients communicate by song. Musical ability is organized on the nondominant hemisphere.

F I G U R E 7-1
The major anatomic areas involved in language.

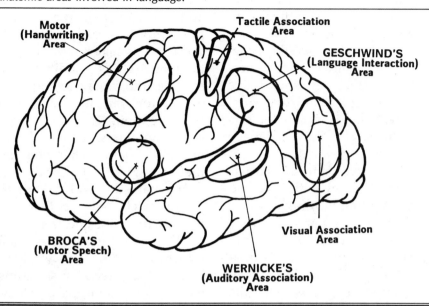

Receptive Dysphasias

Patients in this category have each primary sensory modality intact but cannot use that input for language. For example, one dysphasic patient group can see but cannot read. Another group can hear but cannot comprehend. Patients with a receptive dysphasia cannot convert a primary modality into language code.

Patients with *visual agnosia* can see but cannot name or recognize objects or letters; however, they can occasionally copy letters or objects. Reception of language by any sense entails two steps: first, activation of either the right or left primary sensory cortex; and second, interpretation into language codes of what is seen by the primary sensory cortex.

The interpretation of visual input into language code takes place in the visual association area of the dominant hemisphere (Fig. 7-1). When the letter "A" is shown in your left visual field, the shape is perceived on the right cal-

crine cortex of the occipital lobe (see Fig. 4-19). That shape must be transmitted via the posterior corpus callosum to the visual association area on the left before you can recognize the shape as the letter "A." Patients without a posterior corpus callosum cannot use an object in the left visual field to stimulate language. They are unable to name objects seen in the left visual field, but they can copy them. When objects are presented in the right visual field, they identify them correctly.

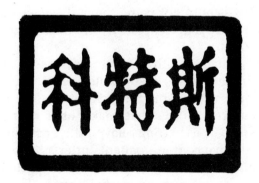

The Chinese ideographs above give us some idea of the problem. We can see them and copy them, but, unless we have studied Chinese, they are without language content for us. We can neither pronounce them nor compare them with any other language experience. If written in English letters, you would recognize them as my name. When pronounced in Chinese, they sound like Curtis. We can complete the first step, perception, but cannot complete the second step, translation into language code.

Patients with visual agnosia can use spoken language, as they both hear and speak fluently. Writing may be impaired because they cannot compare what they write with what they wish to communicate. The lesion is in the visual association area of the dominant (left) hemisphere and leaves patients without the ability to perceive written language even though they can see.

Tactile agnosia has been studied in a few patients with damage to the central part of the corpus callosum. Objects placed in the left hand could be drawn by the left hand but not by the right hand. These patients could not name common shapes placed in their left hands. The information could not cross to the tactile association area of the dominant parietal lobe, where the shape is identified and a language code assigned. As a result, the shapes did not enter the rest of the language system, and patients could not name them. They easily named shapes placed in their right hands.

Patients with *Wernicke's dysphasia*, or verbal agnosia, respond to verbal questions with rapid strings of well-pronounced words that make little or no sense. These strings have little or no intellectual content; patients utter a "word salad." You will see patients with partial lesions who make partial sense. They have great difficulty repeating words or phrases. The phrase "no ifs, ands, or buts" defeats them.

The lesion responsible for Wernicke's dysphasia surrounds the primary auditory cortex on the dominant superior temporal gyrus and is known as the *auditory association area* (Fig. 7-1). Patients with this condition cannot turn sounds into language code for processing or for transmission to Broca's area for repetition. They even have trouble sounding out words. Because they do not understand what you are asking, their answers make little sense. Moreover, patients with Wernicke's dysphasia rarely tell you that they do not understand your question.

Many of these patients have great difficulty reading and writing, perhaps because they read by sounding out the words for themselves. Many normal people actually move their lips and sound out the words as they read. When shown a picture of a chair and asked to identify it, patients with Wernicke's dysphasia may say "chair," use a paraphrase such as "stool," or utter some jargon such as "chassis."

The ability to write the name of an object is usually better preserved in these patients than is the capacity to say the name of an object. Patients with Wernicke's dysphasia can usually follow simple written instructions. Taking a history by writing answers to short questions is time consuming, but it gets the information.

With the advent of computerized tomography (CT) and magnetic resonance imaging (MRI) scanning, we can pinpoint these lesions and even use their size to indicate what types of language therapy may be most helpful.

Cognitive Dysphasias

After receiving sensory symbols and turning them into language codes, we compare those language codes with our experience; we think about the incoming symbols. When confronted with a red octagonal stop sign, we compare that input with our experience and put on the brake. Patients with cognitive dysphasias have difficulty making the connections between sensory association areas and motor areas.

Conduction dysphasia is a condition in which aural comprehension is good, but speech, albeit fluent, makes little sense. Patients with conduction dysphasia are different from those with Wernicke's dysphasia because they can comprehend the spoken request to "place your left hand on your left ear." Patients with conduction dysphasia are different from those with Broca's dysphasia because the former's speech is fluent and their words are understandable. These patients have a lesion in the white matter beneath the central sulcus, near the lateral fissure. This lesion interrupts the large fiber bundle running from the superior temporal gyrus (Wernicke's area) to the inferior frontal area (Broca's area).

Anomia describes the inability to name familiar objects in spite of intact sensory and sensory association areas. The lesion is in the posterior and lateral temporal lobe near the occipital lobe boundary.

Global aphasia inevitably results from lesions to the angular and supermarginal gyri of the dominant parietal lobe (Fig. 7-1). Patients have intact sensory areas but cannot interconnect any of them. Singing is often preserved. I believe these two gyri are the central point of the language system (Fig. 7-1). Here the various inputs merge and are directed to any of the language output areas. I propose we name this area after the person who pointed out its importance; we will call it Geschwind's area. Both gyri are proportionately very large in humans compared with those of other primate brains.

Pure lesions of Geschwind's area are rare because of its close proximity to Wernicke's area just across the lateral fissure. Any space-occupying lesion in the region encompasses both areas, and both are served by the same branch of the middle cerebral artery. The loss of both areas gives almost total loss of language; such loss deserves the name aphasia.

LEFT-HANDEDNESS

About 5% of the population chooses the left hand for fine motor activity, including writing. Motor control of fine motor activity, including handwriting, is in the right frontal lobe; lesions here result in apraxia.

About one-third of all left-handed individuals have a left-dominant (for language) cerebral cortex; left-sided strokes cause the same sorts of problems you would expect in persons who are right-handed. Another one-third have a right-dominant hemisphere. Neither group is, however, as devastated by strokes to the dominant hemisphere as are right-handers. The remaining third have language function in both hemispheres, Broca's area on one side and Wernick's area on the other, for example.

While it is possible to transfer language functions from left to right hemisphere after damage, successful cases have all been in young patients less than 12 years old. Such treatment requires vast effort.

THE NONDOMINANT HEMISPHERE

Anatomically there are minor differences between the two hemispheres but, as yet, cerebral dominance cannot be determined from size alone. Since the hemispheres are roughly the same size, what

F I G U R E 7-2
Increased glucose metabolism when listening to language or music. These are
horizontal sections at the level of the right and left superior temporal gyri. (Traced from
positron emission tomography (PET) scan records in Figure 6-6 of Harbert, J., and Da
Rocha, A. F. G.: *Textbook of Nuclear Medicine,* p. 135. Philadelphia, Lea & Febiger,
1984.)

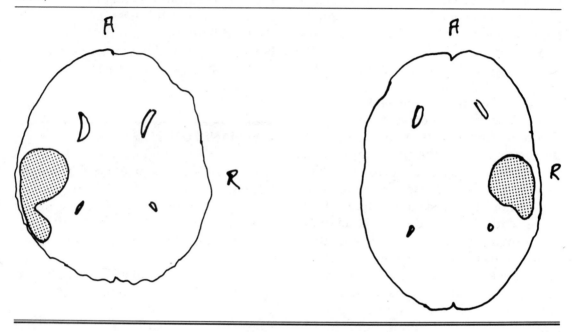

are the higher functions of the non-dominant hemisphere? Music is one. The nondominant hemisphere becomes more active while the subject is listening to music than when the subject is listening to an equivalent amount of speech (Fig. 7-2). Singing is usually preserved in patients with dominant hemisphere strokes. Musicians who have suffered dominant hemisphere strokes may need a musical cue to begin playing but often do so well. Although they can learn new compositions by ear, reading the notes may not be possible. They certainly cannot read the words.

Many patients with strokes in the nondominant hemisphere develop an impatient and impulsive behavior. Their behavior makes recovery from any impairment such as hemiparesis, hemianopsia, or a hemisensory loss much harder than you might expect. Further,

these patients neglect their nondominant side or even ignore its existence. Dressing tends to be very difficult for them. When asked to draw a clock, only the right side will be completed. They only eat from the right side of their plate. Since they "see" only the right side of objects or people, recognition is difficult. They may use a toothbrush on the hair.

MEMORY

The recall of events, words, or pictures can be divided into two stages, short and long term. Most of us can remember, through *short-term memory,* a seven- or ten-digit telephone number for 1 to 3 minutes if we are not overly distracted. Patients can lose short-term auditory memory without losing short-term visual memory. The cortical association areas are the loci for short-term memory.

Some of the our short-term memories are converted into *long-term* (Fig. 7-3). Recall of events, faces, or telephone numbers from hours or years ago comes from long-term memory. The conversion of short-term to long-term memory is very fragile. Unconsciousness causes memory loss for events just before (*retrograde amnesia*) and just after (*anterograde amnesia*) unconsciousness, but memory for events further back in time remains intact. The time span of the memory loss is related to the severity of the injury and may be several months.

Localization of long-term memory storage has proved illusive. Repeated stimulation of the temporal lobe in conscious patients brings back exactly the same specific memory. Excision of the stimulated area, however, does not eradicate the memory. Large areas of the anterior and lateral temporal lobe can be removed without demonstrable long-term memory deficit. Both frontal lobes also play a role in long-term memory.

Patients with bilateral damage to the medial temporal lobes, particularly to the amygdala and hippocampus (Fig. 7-4), cannot inscribe new long-term memory. "Yesterday" was a few weeks or months before the event. I recently talked to a person who was a salesman "yesterday" for DeSoto cars that were last produced in the early 1950s. These patients can function in everyday life only by leaving themselves copious notes of what they intend. Any distraction causes complete loss of the idea of what had been done and what was intended to be done.

The amygdala receives input from all the sensory cortices. Most of the amygdala outflow is to the hippocampus (Fig. 7-4). The hippocampus is in turn connected to the frontal and temporal lobes.

Understanding the memory function of the amygdala and hippocampus is complicated by their role in emotional and instinctive behavior. They belong to a larger group of structures, the *limbic system* (Fig. 7-4). This system includes the cingulate gyrus, the prefrontal areas of the frontal lobe, the mamillary body, and a large fiber tract, called the fornix, that interconnects them. Disease in these structures can fundamentally alter the mood and personality to the extent that these persons cannot pay attention or cooperate.

F I G U R E 7-3
The relation between short-term/long-term memory and language input/output.

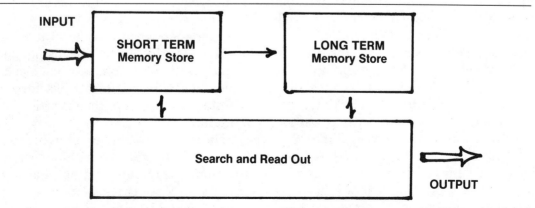

F I G U R E 7-4
The major structures of the limbic system seen in a hemisected brain with the brain stem removed.

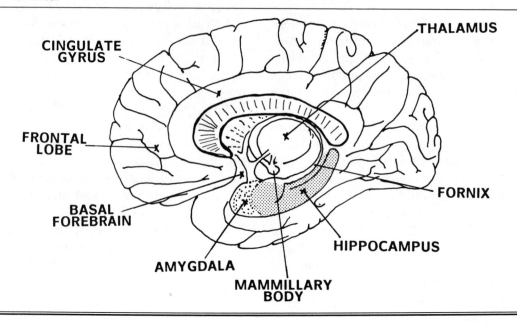

DEMENTIA

We lose nerve cells, especially cerebral cortical neurons, in the normal course of aging. This is most apparent in the converson from short-term to long-term memory. Memory for events that happened long ago remains good. Most of us learn to leave many more notes and reminders as the years go by. Like all biologic events, there is much variability in the rate of loss of the translation from short-term to long-term memory. This loss is sometimes debilitating to a 60-year-old with no apparent disease pathology, while an 80-year-old may be publishing a book a year. Against this background of extreme variability, deciding when a disease process is responsible for memory loss is very difficult.

Dementia is usually defined as intellectual deterioration severe enough to interfere with occupational or social performance. In addition to memory loss, dementia includes the loss of attentive power, shallow and impulsive thought and affect, and emotional lability. New cases of dementia in previously healthy 80-year-olds develop at the rate of 1% to 2% per year, occurring as commonly as myocardial infarction and twice as commonly as stroke.

Transient dementia commonly occurs after an acute illness such as a hip fracture. Older persons may be living alone quite well until a fracture occurs. They then need a great deal of help regaining their independence and, unfortunately, many never do. Emotional insults such as the death of a spouse can have the same effect. The death rate of widowers is almost twice that of their married contemporaries.

There are a number of remediable causes of dementia. Frontal lobe tumors and normal pressure hydrocephalus are examples. Most cases of dementia are caused by widespread disease such as multiple small strokes, particularly in the frontal lobe, or by generalized reduction in blood flow secondary to atherosclerosis. The long latency virus causing Creutzfeldt-Jakob disease is a rare cause of dementia, yet should be considered because of its infectious nature.

Alzheimer's disease is probably caused by several different normal and pathologic processes; all lead to dementia. It is not clear whether the neurofibrillary tangles seen on biopsy or autopsy specimens are causative or merely tomb-

stones of a variety of disease processes. Unfortunately for these patients and their families, the disease progress is downhill. These patients require extraordinary care, usually in an institution.

POST-TEST

The checkered areas are regions of maximal blood flow increase during the stated activity as measured by Xenon 133. For each diagram, determine the

Active areas during language activity

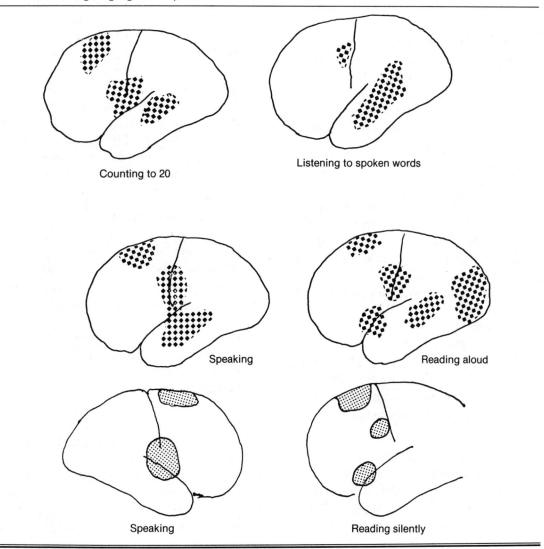

Counting to 20

Listening to spoken words

Speaking

Reading aloud

Speaking

Reading silently

anatomical areas receiving increased flow and speculate upon their function in that activity. (Traced from the work of Lassen, N., Ingar, D., and Skinhoj, E.: *Arch Neurol* 33:523, 1976.)

CASE HISTORIES

1. Ms. A. H., a 76-year-old right-handed woman, fell down a short flight of stairs. Her family tells you she is very healthy and active. When asked simple verbal questions, she responds with clearly pronounced words that do not fit the situation. When asked where it hurts, she replies "Lark." Often she speaks long strings of well-pronounced words that have no meaning. "I when going eat sing." When asked to point to her left ear, she does so. There is a mild weakness of her right face. Handwriting is unsteady.

2. A 28-year-old right-handed woman suffered a stroke 1 week after cesarean section. She responds to spoken questions with short words: "yes," "no," or "maybe." She repeats the short words "dog" and "cat." She pronounces "television" as "teli-bishin" and cannot point to the TV set in the room. When the math problem $(3 \times 4) + 1$ is written out for her, she slowly speaks her way through the problem. "Three times four is twelve and one is thirteen." When the same problem is spoken to her, she cannot repeat it, much less solve it.

3. A 57-year-old right-handed woman suffered a sudden, mild stroke. Mild weakness in the right hand and the right side of the face appeared. During the first week she spoke with long pauses between short words and had difficulty beginning each word. With longer words she made many errors. She could count to 10 very quickly. For the next few weeks she rarely opened a conversation but did respond slowly to questions. She could readily follow three-step commands. Her weak right hand first became spastic, and then strength returned. After extensive speech therapy, she now can use four- and five-syllable words. (Based on a case presented by Tonkonogy and Goodglass: *Arch Neurol* 38:486–490, 1981.)

4. A 37-year-old woman suddenly has difficulty speaking; she seems to know what she wants to say but cannot get it out. She responds to spoken questions with clear, logical written answers. Her speech is hoarse. When asked to stick out her tongue, it deviates to the right and her uvula rises to the left. Her right vocal cord is paralyzed. She has a coarse tremor during finger-to-nose testing.

5. A 66-year-old music professor gave an impressive performance on a four-manual organ during the first part of a concert. During intermission he drank a glass of water, walked to a pew rather than to the organ, and there leafed aimlessly through a hymnal. His wife escorted him to the organ and opened the music to the proper page. He looked blank. She knew something was wrong so she hummed the first line; hearing her voice, "he jumped right in" and played the piece correctly. The recital was then concluded prematurely because she realized he was "sick." He acknowledged the applause in his usual manner. (Based on a case described by Byer, J., and Crowley, W. J.: *Neurology* 30:80–82, 1980.)

C H A P T E R

8

Chemical Neuroanatomy

Chemical neuroanatomy is the study of groups of neurons that release the same neurotransmitter. Just as groups of neurons with common origins and similar destinations have a common function, so we expect a common function of a group of neurons releasing the same neurotransmitter.

Grouping neurons by the neurotransmitter they release is intriguing because synaptic events are readily modulated by drugs. The neuromuscular junction we discussed in Chapter 2 is an example. We can hope to manipulate central nervous system synapses by drug therapy. This is a hope partially sustained by reality. There are perhaps 20 to 30 known neurotransmitters in the central nervous system (CNS).

The first challenge to neuroscientists was to identify neurochemical systems, just as earlier neuroanatomists identified the tracts you learned about in earlier chapters. While the job is not complete, a number of neurochemical systems have been worked out in great detail.

The second challenge to neuroscientists is to match neurochemical systems with specific brain functions. We are on

the threshold of these studies; today we have only some of the pieces of this puzzle and are not sure how they fit together. We currently know more about altered function of neurochemical systems than we do about their normal function. Hence, we will only be able to take a brief look at today's frontier of neuroscience, chemical neuroanatomy and neuropharmacology.

This section describes the neurotransmitter *dopamine* of the *catecholamine* family of neurotransmitters in some detail. Although less than 1% of the brain's neurons use dopamine as a transmitter, dopamine is well localized in three anatomic areas and two functional groups. Anatomically, dopamine is located in the substantia nigra, the caudate and putamen, and the frontal lobe. Functionally, dopamine is involved in a movement disorder, Parkinson's disease, and in a psychosis, schizophrenia.

The Catecholamine Family. To understand dopamine's actions, we need some familiarity with neurochemistry. The catecholamine family of neurotransmitters is based on the essential dietary

F I G U R E 8-1

The catecholamine synthetic pathway. The circled chemical group indicates the transformation carried out. The enzymes are TH, tyrosine hydroxylase (TH); dopa decarboxylase (DDC); dopamine β-hydroxylase (DBH); and phenylethanolamine-N-methyltransferase (PNMT).

amino acid *tyrosine* (Fig. 8-1). The enzyme tyrosine hydroxylase (TH) creates a second hydroxyl (OH) group on the ring structure, thereby producing Dopa. The enzyme TH is the rate-controlling step of the pathway. Control systems inhibit the enzyme and prevent further conversion of tyrosine. Inhibition of the enzyme controls the amount of neurotransmitter stored in a neuron terminal.

Dopa is rapidly converted to dopamine. In many neurons the catecholamine synthetic pathway ends here, and dopamine is packaged into presynaptic vesicles. These vesicles release dopamine from axon terminals when action potentials come from the cell body.

A few central and all peripheral neurons of the sympathetic nervous system convert dopamine to *norepinephrine* (noradrenaline). Norepinephrine is also packaged in presynaptic vesicles for release and is a potent neurotransmitter. The adrenal medulla transforms norepinephrine into *epinephrine* (adrenaline) for release into the bloodstream.

DOPAMINE SYSTEM

Just as some neurons package dopamine into vesicles for release when the neuron is activated, there are also cells that have *dopamine receptors* on their surface. These receptors bind dopamine. The dopamine-receptor complex alters either a membrane event or an intercellular process in the postsynaptic neuron.

There are two major types of dopamine receptors, D_1 and D_2. When activated by binding with dopamine, the D_1 receptor stimulates production of an intercellular messenger, cyclic adenosine monophosphate (cAMP), within the cell. For many minutes after activation, cAMP modifies cell behavior. Just what increased cAMP concentrations do inside a cell depends on which enzymes and channels have been expressed from the cell's DNA genome. D_1 receptor activation may stimulate one neuron yet inhibit another neuron with a different set of intracellular machinery.

When activated by dopamine, D_2 receptors inhibit cAMP production. Depending on the particular cell, activation of D_2 receptor by dopamine leads to a variety of cellular responses.

Specific exciters (*agonists*) and specific blockers (*antagonists*) for both D_1 and D_2 receptors have been developed. Our ability to synthesize compounds in the laboratory that have chemical structures very similar to dopamine, but with differences in action, is the basis of pharmacologic specificity. For example, a D_2 antagonist blocks the effect of liberated dopamine on cells with D_2 receptors, while cells with D_1 receptors bind dopamine and respond by increasing production of cAMP.

Once released from presynaptic vesicles, dopamine binds to postsynaptic receptors and is slowly removed from the synaptic junction. About 80% is removed by uptake into nerve terminals and about 20% is inactivated by the enzyme monoamine oxydase.

Nigro-Striatal System

Some 80% of the dopamine-containing neurons lie within the basal ganglia. These neurons run from the substantia nigra of the midbrain (see Fig. 4-18) to the caudate and putamen, which jointly are called the *corpus striatum* (see Figs. 5-10 and 5-12). The nigro-striatal system branches widely; one neuron in the substantia nigra influences upward of 500,000 neurons in the corpus striatum. Consequently, the striatum contains far higher concentrations of dopamine than does the substantia nigra.

This nigro-striatal dopamine system inhibits the action of the striatum. Dopamine counters an excitatory function in the striatum transmitted by acetylcholine-releasing neurons. The dopamine and acetylcholine systems act in opposition, much as the gas pedal and the brake act in a car.

Parkinson's Disease. Parkinson's disease, the shaking palsy, begins with *akinesia*, that is, a reduction of spontaneous movement. At first, the akinesia is very subtle but becomes more pronounced with time. When resting tremors are noticed, patients usually seek help. Finally, rigidity begins and slowly becomes debilitating. The disease is usually first diagnosed in patients in their mid-50s and slowly progresses over the next 5 to 10 years. Without treatment, the underlying akinesia and rigidity slowly disable these patients until they need continuous care. There are a number of recognized variants of Parkinson's disease.

The basic pathology of Parkinson's disease is a loss of substantia nigra cells, including the pigment-containing cells (Fig. 8-2). Since these dopamine neurons project to the striatum, there is a dramatic loss of dopamine in the corpus striatum (Fig. 8-3). The cause of this cellular loss is unknown.

Once scientists learned that a dopamine deficiency is the underlying pathophysiology of the disease, attempts at dopamine replacement began. Because dopamine does not cross the blood-brain barrier, replacement therapy is with its precursor, dopa. Extracellular dopa is somehow converted into dopamine, or acts as a dopamine agonist, once it crosses into the synaptic regions of the striatum. Whatever its mechanism, dopa is effective in altering corpus striatum function.

Many patients have a 50% or greater improvement in their rigidity and akinesia in the first few months of therapy.

FIGURE 8-2

Depigmentation of the substantia nigra of a Parkinson's patient (*left*) in contrast to that of a normal patient (*right*). (Courtesy of Uma Kalyan-Raman, M.D., University College of Medicine at Peoria, IL.)

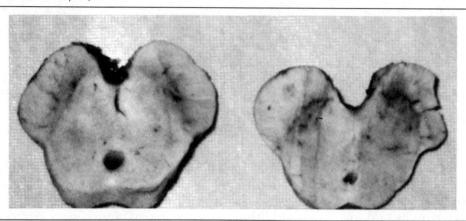

This improvement slowly wanes over the next few years but is still appreciable after 10 years. Dopa's therapeutic effects are unlikely to be specific effects on specific neurons. It is much more likely that the neurons of the striatum are awash in a sea of neurotransmitters. The neurotransmitters dopamine and acetylcholine set the general level of activity of the striatum. To return to the car analogy, a

FIGURE 8-3

A positron emission tomography (PET) scan using radioactive dopa as the tracer. In normal persons (**A**), the corpus striatum takes up the tracer at high levels (*stippled area*). In patients with Parkinson's disease (**B**), the uptake is much reduced. (Traced from color illustrations in Goetz, C. G., Jankovic, J., and Paulson, G. W.: *Patient Care,* April 15, 1989.

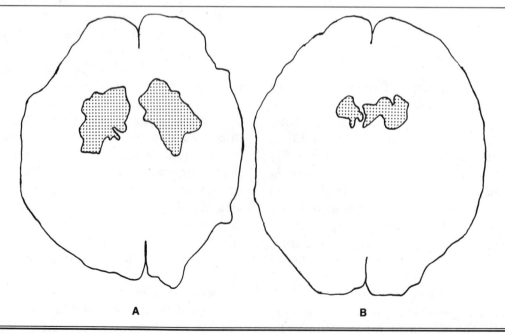

A   B

car's speed is determined by the balance between the gas pedal and the brake.

Drug Therapy. Dopa or levodopa (Larodopa) is widely used in the treatment of Parkinson's disease. Ingested dopa is distributed to both the brain and the body. To prevent dopa-to-dopamine conversion in the body, an inhibitor of the conversion of dopa to dopamine is given concomitantly. Hence, dopa conversion to dopamine is suppressed in the body and dopa plasma levels remain high. Dopa conversion to dopamine in the brain is normal because the conversion inhibitor cannot cross the blood-brain barrier. The commonly used preparation in the treatment of Parkinson's disease (Sinemet) is a combination of dopa and carbidopa, a dopa-conversion inhibitor.

Several other drugs are useful in Parkinson's disease therapy. Amantadine (Symmetrel) causes release of dopamine from both central and peripheral presynaptic terminals and has proved useful. Bromocriptine (Parlodel), a dopamine agonist, is sometimes useful. Selegiline (Deprenyl) inhibits monoamine oxydase, the enzyme that destroys dopamine; selegiline consequently keeps the naturally released dopamine in the synaptic region longer, which enhances neurotransmission.

Anticholinergic drugs are sometimes useful in reducing the stimulatory effects of the cholinergic system in the corpus striatum. This treatment brings the cholinergic system more into balance with the diminished capacity of the dopamine system, an inhibitory system. Its use is analogous to making up for poor brakes by using low-octane gas.

All these drugs are effective in treating neurochemical imbalances but do not treat the underlying disease. The cause of Parkinson's disease is unknown. Diagnosis of the disease's subtypes and the choice of an appropriate treatment regime require great clinical skill.

Recent attempts to transplant dopamine-secreting cells into the caudate nucleus have been the subject of numerous newspaper articles but have had mixed medical success. Enough success has been achieved, however, to ensure continued efforts along these lines.

The Mesocortical System

The remaining 20% of the dopamine system runs from the midbrain and ends diffusely in both cingulate gyri. The cingulate gyri set a person's general behavioral outlook and are part of the limbic system (see Fig. 7-4). Drugs acting on the dopamine system have proved useful in the treatment of mental illness and are thought to have their action on the mesocortical dopamine system.

Schizophrenia. Schizophrenia describes a group of personality disorders, or acute psychoses, that begin between 15 and 35 years of age. Schizophrenia is characterized by positive symptoms such as hallucinations and delusions and by negative symptoms such as withdrawal and introversion. In general, positive symptoms respond more readily to drug therapy than do the negative ones.

Many theories have been proposed to explain the neurochemical basis of schizophrenia, but the longest-lasting theory proposes an excess of dopaminergic activity in the mesocortical circuit. We currently understand so little about the structural and neurochemical basis of behavior that no explanation can be given of how personality is changed by excess dopamine activity. We are searching for clues; here are some of them.

All neuroleptic drugs useful in the amelioration of schizophrenia bind to dopamine receptors but do not activate them. Instead, these drugs prevent activation by dopamine. The most useful drugs block only the D_2 receptors in the limbic system. There is a very close parallel between dopamine receptor-binding studies in animals and the drug's potency as an antipsychotic in humans.

Several drugs useful in treating schizophrenia have left-handed versions that bind to D_2 receptors and right-handed versions that do not bind; only the left-handed versions are effective neuroleptics. Positron emission tomography (PET) studies show a reduction of dopamine binding in the human striatum after neuroleptic drug therapy; the neuroleptics have covered up, but not activated, the dopamine receptor sites. Unfortunately, the D_2 receptor concentration in the cingulate gyri is too low to be detectable with current PET methods. There seems to be little doubt that neuroleptic drugs bind to and block D_2 receptors and that their effectiveness relates to this binding.

Postmortem neurochemical studies on schizophrenic patients show a doubling of the number of D_2 receptors in the mesolimbic system. It would seem that a greater than normal number of D_2-receptor proteins were expressed from the DNA genome. There is some evidence of a genetic component to schizophrenia; a child of two schizophrenics has a 40% greater chance of affliction than a child of nonafflicted parents.

Several other observations point to an increased dopaminergic transmission as a cause of schizophrenia. Amphetamines stimulate release of dopamine from nerve terminals and often induce a schizophrenic-like psychosis. About 15% of patients treated with dopa develop schizophrenic side effects and have to be taken off the medication. Not surprisingly, the common side effects of neuroleptic drugs resemble the rigidity and akinesia seen in Parkinson's disease.

Drug Therapy. A number of enigmas remain concerning schizophrenia. A general reduction in cortical blood flow and glucose metabolism is seen in PET scans of schizophrenics. This reduction is certainly not limited to the frontal lobe. This generalized reduction in blood flow returns to normal with effective drug therapy.

The phenothiazine family of drugs are dopamine antagonists that have revolutionized the treatment of mental disorders including schizophrenia. Among the most used are chlorpromazine (Thorazine), molindone hydrochloride (Moban), and haloperidol (Haldol).

We have a great deal more to learn about chemical neuroanatomy and its relation to brain function. It is clear that major advances in the treatment of CNS disease will come from these studies.

POST-TEST

1. What are the characteristics of the presynaptic region?

2. What are the characteristics of the synaptic cleft?

3. What are the characteristics of the postsynaptic region?

4. Neurotransmitters are identified by what four criteria?

5. What system controls the amount of dopamine stored in the presynaptic region?

6. What is the intercellular action of an activated D_1 receptor?

7. If a synapse is first treated with a D_2 antagonist such as haloperidol, what intercellular response can we expect to release dopamine?

8. What are the major anatomic structures close to the substantia nigra?

9. What structures receive input from the substantia nigra? What is their function?

10. Parkinson's disease is defined by what three symptoms?

11. Why is IV dopamine ineffective in the treatment of Parkinson's disease?

12. Why is carbidopa, a dopa conversion inhibitor, added to the common preparations of dopa?

9

Neuroimaging

METHODS

This chapter is a very brief and, of necessity, superficial introduction to the imaging methods that have revolutionized study and diagnosis of the nervous system. Regular x-ray films (plain films) are still useful for studying the bony skull and vertebral column. X-ray films of blood vessels filled with radiopaque dye (angiograms) continue to be very helpful (see Figs. 5-4, 5-5, and 5-20). Angiography of diseased blood vessels can be combined with intravascular intervention to treat the problem. Examples include compressing atherosclerotic plaque or coagulating aneurysms.

Computed Tomography

Computed tomographpy (CT) uses a narrow beam of x-rays from a rotating x-ray source (Fig. 9-1). The narrow x-ray beam passes through a patient's head and the intensity of the emerging x-ray beam is measured by a detector. The detector rotates together with the x-ray generator.

This method depends on a complex computer program that takes the x-ray absorption of hundreds of x-ray paths through the head and figures out the exact location of the structures absorbing the x-rays. There are two stippled areas in Figure 9-1. The area in the center of rotation absorbs x-rays at every rotational position of the x-ray generator and detector. The other stippled area absorbs x-rays when the beam is in the very limited region centered on the dashed line. A computer program figures out which area is which and generates an absorption map. Regions that absorb x-rays, such as bone, appear light while those that do not, such as the ventricular system, appear dark.

The bony skull absorbs most of the x-rays, and it appears white on CT scans. The structures of the brain have variable x-ray absorption. Cerebral spinal fluid is a particularly poor absorber of x-rays and shows up dark; hence, the ventricles show up well on CT scans. The lateral ventricles are symmetrical structures (see Fig. 5-18). Any deviation from their symmetrical locations suggests a space-occupying lesion.

F I G U R E 9-1
The CT scanner obtains an image by passing a thin beam of x-rays through the head and measuring the intensity of the x-ray beam as it emerges. Both x-ray generator an x-ray detector rotate together to obtain hundreds of data points for each 0.7-cm slice of the brain. A computer program determines the most likely location of the structures doing the absorbing (such as the two stippled areas) and generates the anatomic scans we view.

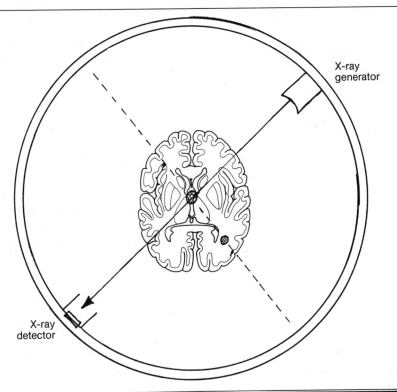

As coagulated blood is an especially good absorber of x-rays, hemorrhages show up well (see Fig. 5-6), as does blood in the subarachnoid space.

Iodide strongly absorbs x-rays and can be incorporated into compounds that do not cross the blood-brain barrier. These contrast-enhancing compounds do not enter healthy brain but do enter most tumors and make the tumor visible on CT scan.

The data from a 0.7-cm slice of the brain can be gathered in 2 to 3 seconds. During this time the patient must be absolutely still. The beam then moves to obtain the data for another slice. Usually 13 to 15 slices are sufficient to image the brain. Advantages of CT scanning in-

clude its rapid completion time and its relatively low cost ($500 in 1989). The dose of x-rays and the poor rendition of structures in the posterior fossa are among its disadvantages.

Magnetic Resonance Imaging

In magnetic resonance imaging (MRI) of the brain, the patient's head is placed into a very strong magnetic field. The magnetic field causes all the hydrogen atoms in the head to orient in the same direction. Short pulses of radio waves are sent through the head and try to upset this orientation. When the radio waves are successful in rearranging the individual hydrogen atoms, the hydrogen atoms give off an electromagnetic signal when the radio wave pulse ends. The electromagnetic signal is usually divided into two parts, an early T_1 signal and a late T_2 signal. The relative magnitudes of the T_1 and T_2 signals give information about the type of tissue emitting the signal.

A computer system maps the location of the electromagnetic wave emission and generates the MRI scans we view. Scans from the T_1 signal define the anatomy of the central nervous system with stunning clarity. In general, the T_2 signal highlights edema, tumors, and other abnormal tissue. Water generates both T_1 and T_2 signals, while bone is a very poor signal generator. Flowing blood generates no signal, so MRI scans show satisfactory black images of blood vessels. Stagnant and decomposed blood gives white images. Contrast agents such as gadolinium are becoming available (see Fig. 4-12).

This method uses no ionizing radiation and is currently thought to be harmless. The only drawbacks to MRI scanning are the longer time needed, (3–5 minutes per exposure), the high cost ($1,000 in 1989), and the claustrophobia that many patients experience while the scan is being done.

The plane of section of the MRI scans in this book are shown in Figure 9-2.

Positron Emission Tomography

Positron emission tomography (PET) relies on a radioisotope injected into the body. The radioisotope emits a positron that collides with a nearby electron. The collision produces two x-rays that fly off in opposite directions to be captured by a ring of detectors around the head (Fig. 9-3). A computer puts the origin of the x-rays onto a map and generates the scans.

F I G U R E 9-2
A synopsis of the MRI sections in this book.

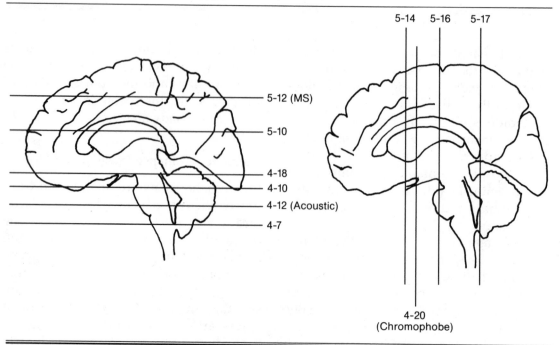

F I G U R E 9-3
A radioisotope localized to the caudate gives off a positron that collides with an
electron and generates two x-rays that head off in opposite directions. These x-rays are
captured by a ring of detectors. A computer program generates the PET scan we view

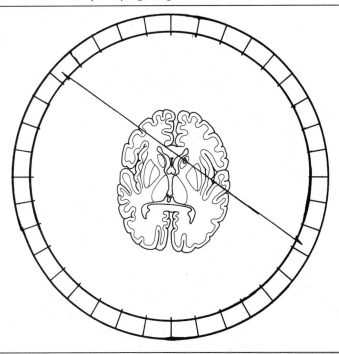

The radioisotope can be incorporated into a variety of compounds. To study blood flow to regions of the brain, the radioisotope used is O^{15}. To study metabolism, the radioisotope F^{17} is hooked to glucose. The radioactive compound can be neurochemically important (see Fig. 8-3). We can learn a great deal about normal brain function as well as dysfunction in disease from PET scanning.

This method uses very low doses of radiation. Its major drawback is its very great expense ($3,000 per study in 1989). It is largely a research tool in the CNS.

Case Histories

Elliott Marcus, M.D.

In the case histories that follow, first attempt to isolate the lesion to a single level of the nervous system or to a fiber system by using the clues of functions both lost and retained. In some of these cases, you may decide, based on the history and findings, that multiple levels of the nervous system are involved. Then use the clues of the history and location of the lesion to speculate on the type of disease causing the deficits. What further diagnostic studies are called for? What are the therapeutic options?

Case 1. A 63-year-old right-handed bartender has lost weight, has been fatigued, and has had changes in bowel habits for the last few months. Two weeks ago he began having spontaneous twitching of the left corner of his mouth associated with a tingling sensation in his left tumb and index finger. These last 1 to 2 minutes and have been happening once or twice a day. There has been no loss of consciousness and no generalized convulsion.

These case histories have been adapted from *An Introduction to the Neurosciences.*

On examination there is a flattening of the left nasolabial fold. The left side of his mouth does not pull back well, giving him a lopsided smile. Deep tendon reflexes in the left arm are hyperactive. Stereognosis and graphesthesia are impaired in the left hand.

Case 2. Seven years ago a 59-year-old plumbing contractor noted the onset of a tremor of his right hand occurring mainly at rest. There was no loss of strength or sensation in the right hand. A year ago the tremor was also present at the wrist and shoulder.

On examination, the patient is depressed and anxious with a mild impairment of delayed recall and ability to retell stories. His face is fixed and without associated movements when he talks. He rarely changes posture although his strength is intact. He walks with slow, short steps and turns with a shuffling *en bloc* motion. There is a resting tremor of his right arm and fingers. The right arm and leg show resistance to passive motion with a cogwheel component at the right shoulder, elbow, and wrist.

Case 3. A 53-year-old homemaker noted the onset of weakness and "twitching" in the muscles of her left leg about 1 month ago. She has been feeling fatigued and lethargic for some time but remains alert without any change in mental status.

The muscles of her left leg are atrophied and widespread fasciculations are present. Both left knee and ankle reflexes are absent. Sensation is everywhere normal.

Case 4. Two months ago, a 45-year-old male had a transient episode of left facial weakness and difficulty remembering names. At that time his serum cholesterol was 332 mg/dl (normal < 160 mg/dl). This morning he awoke with numbness on the left side of his face and tongue. Diplopia was present, particularly on looking to the left. When he arose from bed, he noted vertigo and walked with a staggering gait.

On examination several hours later he has a left lateral rectus weakness and an intention tremor of his left hand. The numbness of his left face and tongue is rapidly disappearing. Speech is slurred. There is an intention tremor of his left hand with impairment of alternating movements.

Case 5. For the past week, a 42-year-old bookkeeper has had severe headaches that have not responded to aspirin. She reports having trouble with her eyes for some time. For 20 years she has had thyroid difficulty that has not responded to thyroid medication. Her menses ceased when she was 20. During the past few years she has had a number of automobile accidents, particularly involving cars coming from her right. During the previous month she has felt excessively tired and has been sleeping more than usual, but has continued to go to work. Her skin is dry, she has

gradually put on weight over the years, and her hair is very thin.

Her visual fields show a bitemporal, upper quadratic field defect with a bilateral pallor of the optic disks.

Case 6. A 69-year-old retired assembly line worker has had three or more episodes of weakness of his right hand, usually with clumsiness and numbness. The most recent episode, which he reports as being the worst, occurred earlier this morning when his right leg also felt weak for the first time. The weakness and numbness have cleared in a few minutes each time, but the clumsiness has lingered for several hours. In the last 2 months he has had three episodes of monocular blindness in his left eye that have been of 3-minute duration. He has had diabetes mellitus for approximately 20 years, which has been treated sporadically with oral antihyperglycemic medication.

There is a bruit in the left neck, and light pressure on the left eyeball leads to a blackout of vision. Deep tendon reflexes are increased in the right arm and decreased in both ankles. There is a mild decrease in vibration sensation in both ankles and wrists. Letter and number recognition in the right hand (graphesthesia) was mildly impaired.

Case 7. An 80-year-old man has had increasing weakness of his legs for the past few months. Thirteen years ago he had a prostatectomy. Ten years ago he had replacement of the right femoral artery by a graft. He has had poor bladder control for several months. About 3 weeks ago he noticed unsteadiness of gait with his right leg worse than the left. This morning he was suddenly weak in both legs.

He is moderately disoriented for time, but he is oriented for place. He provided a coherent history but the actual dates were somewhat vague. There is a mild nominal aphasia. Strength is intact in both arms with bilateral grasp reflexes. There is a tremor when his arms are outstretched. Both legs show spastic weakness with hyperreflexia and bilateral Babinski's signs. He cannot walk. He cannot feel pinprick below the xiphoid process bilateral. Position sense is absent at the left toe and ankle. He is incontinent of both bowel and bladder. There was tenderness over the T7 and T8 spinous processes.

Case 8.   A 23-year-old right-handed army recruit was evaluated at sick call yesterday with an apparent upper respiratory infection and was given a day of barracks rest. At reveille, he was found in his bed, unresponsive. He could not be roused; he had been incontinent of bladder and bowels.

He has a temperature of 103°F, blood pressure of 130/70, and a pulse of 96. He has a diffuse rash with a number of ecchymotic areas. He is in a coma although his extremities withdraw in the presence of painful stimuli. There is marked nuchal rigidity. The pupils are in midposition and respond poorly to light. White blood count was markedly elevated (42,000) with 64% neutrophils, 31% bands, and 5% lymphocytes.

Case 9.   A 62-year-old divorcee has had a personality and memory change. She had a high school education and had been described previously as a bright, alert, and intelligent woman. She cannot provide a history and has no insight into her problem. Her son stated she began to show some decline in intellectual capacity as long as 3 or 4 years ago. In the preceding year the changes have been more marked, particularly her declining memory. In the last few months she has been indifferent to her personal appearance. She has lost interest in her home, friends, and activities.

She is unable to remember any of four test objects after a 5-minute period. She cannot remember the year she was born. She is unable to recall any president but the current one. She is able to follow very simple directions but unable to remember them for 5 minutes.

Case 10.   A 44-year-old married machine operator noted a general sense of fatigue in his arms and legs at the end of the day for several years. The weakness became more marked 6 or 7 weeks ago and occurred in the mornings as well. When chewing, his jaw would become weak. His speech has become slurred and he has difficulty swallowing. Because his eyelids droop, he has difficulty driving. None of these last three symptoms are present initially in the morning.

He has bilateral ptosis that increases markedly with repetitive blinking and bilateral facial weakness that worsens on repeated smiling. Jaw and tongue movements are weak. Both his arms and hands are weak, but reflexes are normal.

Case 11.   A week ago a 51-year-old car saleswoman developed episodic posterior headaches beginning in the neck and radiating to the vortex of the head. Aspirin afforded little relief. The headaches were usually related to and definitely exacerbated by straining or coughing. She noticed clumsiness of her left hand and a tendency to fall to the left side. All her symptoms have progressed in the last week. Six months ago she was treated for an infiltrative and anaplastic carcinoma of the uterine cervix.

She has a coarse nystagmus on gaze to the left. There is a minor dysarthria for lingual and guttural sounds. Strength is intact, but gait is unstable with a tendency to fall to the left, especially when turning to the left. There is marked ataxia on finger-to-nose and heel-to-shin testing.

Case 12. A 21-year-old Air Force–enlisted woman has recently been reassigned away from her husband. She has been complaining of increasingly severe right frontal-temporal or bifrontal headaches for 3 or 4 weeks. During the last 10 days she has been treated at the base dispensary with a variety of medications for an upper respiratory infection or sinusitis. The headaches are now accompanied by blurring of vision and vomiting. The last 48 hours she has been increasingly confused and ataxic.

She is disoriented for time, place, and person and is unable to cooperate with the examination. She is dehydrated and somewhat lethargic with a severe headache, particularly on moving her head. She has bilateral papilledema, and her pupils are dilated and respond slowly to light. She has a left central facial weekness.

Case 13. A 38-year-old right-handed, warehouse manager was in excellent health until yesterday morning when he suddenly lost consciousness. He was found on the floor by his wife who witnessed a generalized convulsive seizure lasting approximately 10 minutes. When he regained consciousness, he had a severe generalized headache and pain in his neck. Because of persistent headaches, he has come in for evaluation.

He is restless and lethargic and has a severe headache. He has marked nuchal rigidity. His neurologic examination was otherwise normal.

Case 14. Two years ago, when she was 26, a right-handed actress noted the onset of numbness of her left leg and a tendency to veer to the left when walking. These symptoms gradually subsided over a period of 7 months. Shortly after the birth of her first child, these symptoms returned, and she had urinary incontinence without the sensation of a full bladder. Bed wetting was frequent. Subsequently she developed vertigo, ataxia, and a clumsiness of the left hand.

She has pallor of the temporal half of the right optic disc, diplopia, and nystagmus on gaze to the right or left. Speech was dysarthric and scanning. Gait was ataxic. An intention tremor was present in the left hand. Bilateral Babinski's signs were present. Position and vibration sensation were absent in the left foot.

Case 15. Approximately 7 or 8 months ago, a 49-year-old right-handed man began to have episodes characterized by a raising sensation beginning at the epigastrium, which lasted 45 to 60 seconds and culminated in an inability to speak or even utter a sound. At this time he would be unable to understand the speech of others. This impairment of language function would last for a minute or so and then clear. These episodes would occur three to five times a week. On some occasions, when he was driving, he would note a change in the appearance of the roadway. The road would appear desolate, empty, or strange and unfamiliar. This sensation of unfamiliarity would pass in a few minutes. He thinks his personality has changed in the last few months. He is depressed at times, cheerful at other times; he has been losing interest in his activities.

He is alert, oriented, and anxious. Physical examination is within normal limits.

R E F E R E N C E S

GENERAL

Books presenting a more comprehensive discussion of the structure and function of the human nervous system include the following:

Brodal, A.: *Neurological Anatomy in Relation to Clinical Medicine* 3rd ed. New York, Oxford University Press, 1981.

Carpenter, M. B., and Sutin, J.: *Human Neuroanatomy*, 8th ed. Baltimore, Williams & Wilkins, 1983.

Marcus, E. M., Jacobson, S., and Curtis, B. A.: *An Introduction to the Neurosciences*. 2nd ed. Philadelphia, Lea & Febiger, 1990.

Peele, R.: *The Neuroanatomical Basis for Clinical Neurology*. New York, McGraw Hill, 1977.

For a colorful review:

Netter, F. H.: *The CIBA collection: Nervous System*. West Caldwell, NJ, CIBA, 1983.

For greater discussion of clinical topics:

Rowland, L. P.: *Merritt's Textbook of Neurology*, 8th ed. Philadelphia, Lea & Febiger, 1989.

Adams, R. D., and Victor, M.: *Principles of Neurology*. 4th ed. New York, McGraw Hill, 1989.

Scientific American and *Science* frequently have well-illustrated articles on the structure and function of the brain.

CHAPTER 2: Nerve and Muscle

Andreoli, T. E., Hoffman, J. F., Fanestil, D. D., and Schultz, S. G.: *Physiology of Membrane Disorders*. New York, Plenum Publishing Corp., 1986.

Brumback, R. A., and Gerst, J. W.: *The Neuromuscular Junction*. Mt. Kisco, NY, Futura, 1984.

Lindstrom, J., Schoepfer, R., and Whiting, P.: Molecular studies on the neuronal nicotinic acetylcholine receptor family. *Mol Neurobiol* 1:281, 1987.

Hille, B.: *Ionic Channels of Excitable Membranes*. Sunderland, MA, Sinauer Associates, Inc., 1984.

Peachey, L. D., and Adrian, R. H.: Sect. 10: Skeletal muscle. *Handbook of Physiology*. Bethesda, MD, American Physiological Society, 1983.

Stein, W. D.: *The Ion Pumps*. New York, Alan R. Liss, Inc., 1988.

CHAPTER 3: Spinal Cord

Brobeck, J.: *Handbook of Physiology*, Section 1. Bethesda, MD, American Physiology Society, 1977.

Davidoff, R. A.: *Handbook of the Spinal Cord*. New York, Marcel Dekker, Inc., 1984.

CHAPTER 4: Brain Stem

Samii, M., and Janetta, P. J.: *The Cranial Nerves*. New York, Springer-Verlag, 1980.

CHAPTER 5: Cerebrum

Jobe, P., and Laird, H.: *Neurotransmitters and Epilepsy*. Humana, 1987.

Portenoy, R. K.: *Pain: Mechanisms and Syndromes*. Neurologic Clinics, Vol. 7, No. 2. Philadelphia, W. B. Saunders, 1989.

Raskin, N. H.: *Headache*. Ed. 2, New York, Churchill-Livingstone, 1988.

Toole, J. F.: *Cerebrovascular Disorders*. New York, Raven Press, 1984.

CHAPTER 6: Movement

Brookhart, J.: Section 1: The Nervous System. *Handbook of Physiology*. Bethesda, MD, American Physiological Society, 1977.

Brooks, V. B.: *The Neural Basis of Motor Control*. New York, Oxford, 1986.

CHAPTER 7: Language and Memory

Bradshaw, J. L., and Nettleton, N. C.: *Human Cerebral Asymmetry*. Englewood Cliffs, NJ, Prentice-Hall, Inc., 1983.

Geschwind, N. and Galaburda, A. M.: Cerebral lateralization. *Arch Neurol* 42:428–459, 1985.

Heilman, K. M., Bowers, T., Valenstein, E., and Watson, R. T.: The right hemisphere: Neuropsychological functions *J Neurosurg* 64:693–704, 1984.

Kandel, E. R.: *Cellular Basis of Behavior*. San Francisco, Freeman, 1976.

Squire, L. R. *Memory and Brain*. New York, Oxford University Press, 1987.

CHAPTER 8: Chemical Neuroanatomy

McGeer, P. L., Eccles, J. C., and McGeer, E. G.: *Molecular Neurobiology of the Mammalian Brain*. New York, Plenum Publishing Corp., 1987.

Snyder, S. H.: Brainstorming: the science and politics of opiate research. Cambridge, MA, Harvard University Press, 1989.

CHAPTER 9: Neuroimaging

Battistein, L., and Gerstenbrand, F.: *PET and MNR*. New York, Alan R. Liss, Inc., 1986.

de Groot, J.: *Magnetic Resonance Imaging*. Philadelphia, Lea & Febiger 1984.

Index